This book is dedicated to all of those who have loved and supported me in my awakening process.

TABLE OF CONTENTS

SESSION WORK

HEALING MODALITIES & CRYSTALS

POTPOURRI

DISCLAIMER

The healing crystals and products offered for sale by the author are not in themselves alleged to be a cure for any ailment, disorder or physical condition. Furthermore, it is not the intention of the author or the publisher to prescribe for any conditions, physical or otherwise. The manner in which this material is interpreted and used is the sole responsibility of the reader. We do recommend that you be involved in a well balanced diet and seek appropriate medical care as needed.

ACKNOWLEDGEMENTS

I wish to acknowledge the following beings for their inspiration or sharing of wisdom along my path of enlightenment: The Ascended Masters Jesus the Christ, St. Germain and Kuthumi. I also would like to thank my spiritual teacher, Sá die who has guided me well. Thank you also to my teachers and friends: Brenda Macaluso; Reiki Master, Patricia Ewing; MariEl Master, Ethel Lombardi; Rev. Margie Laird; Reiki Master, Carol Vidula Krum and recently, Reiki Grandmaster, Phyllis Lei Furumoto.

I also wish to thank the following crystal teachers for their sharing: Fred Rubenfield, Dael Walker, Phillip " Light Bear " McKissick, and Dr. Frank Alper. I thank also the Native American teachers Dhyani Ywahoo and Oh Shinnah for reconnecting me to the Four Directions. Lastly, I'd like to thank the mystery soul who gave me my first crystal in the 1970's. I also would like to thank Mother Earth for her beautiful mountains and the Black Hills of South Dakota. The beauty and energy of these many special places have influenced me with the mineral kingdom since childhood.

It is my friend and assistant, Pat Cade, R.N. who helped to make this book possible. She has been a great catalyst for my coming up with these healing meditations for her and my students. I remember when I first met her and she had asked, " How do you get off on these rocks? " Now, after taking a few classes on crystals and working with their energies over the past couple of years; Pat joins me in applying the use of crystals for healing. I also thank her for using her sensitivity in helping in the evaluation of these meditations and exercises.

I also want to thank Faith Quemen from Newark, Dela. who got me interested in the active meditation techniques of Guided Imagery and Creative Visualization. If I had not taken her weekly classes, this book and these meditations would never have been sparked.

I wish to also thank my eternal soulmate, Eugene Frank for putting up with my insane schedules. It is a blessing to have his full support as my helpmate and companion.

Thank you Susun Weed, for your insight on book publishing and herbs.

I wish to thank Eugene Frank and Dorian Caruso for their assistance in editing this book.

Thanks also goes to Ernie Chu, who in my eleventh hour manifested a word processor.

My greatest crystal teachers have been the crystals themselves. I thank them for their sharing.

PREFACE

Crystals and gemstones have been used throughout ancient civilizations for healing, meditating, protecting and intuitive awakening. Native Americans currently use quartz crystals and specific stones for their healing and meditation work and have done so for centuries. Many books have been written about the energy qualities of quartz crystals and their use. You will find a list at the back of this book for suggested reading. More and more people are becoming curious and interested in crystals. It is all a part of the coming into a New Age.

The purpose of this book is to share with you how I have come to use crystals in my meditations and healing practice. Many of the following exercises have come from meditation, working on clients, or sharing with my students.

I have left some empty pages in this book for you to write down your ideas and impressions. Also, as you take part in these exercises and meditations, you will in turn activate your own healing process and many of you will come up with your own meditations! I hope this book becomes your book as well as my book.

Some of the Crystal Meditations are offered with a list of crystals and gemstones that are suggested with each experience. If you have difficulty in locating crystals and gemstones in your area, feel free to write to us. We carry the most popular items used in the healing arts and at low, reasonable prices. See address at the back of the book.

If you have any questions about these Crystal Healing Meditations, or you would just like to share your experiences feel free to write to me. I will try to answer all inquiries.

We travel and offer training programs in Crystal Therapeutics throughout the country. If you are interested in these programs, or would like us to do seminars in your area, let us know.

May these Crystal Healing Meditations serve to enlighten and heal you as they have for my clients, students and myself.

In Light, Love and Service,

Rev. Ojela Frank

Rev. Ojela Frank

QUARTZ CRYSTALS

Quartz crystals are made up of one part silicon and two parts oxygen; which is also known as, silicon dioxide. Quartz crystals were formed over two hundred million years ago. They are six sided or hexagonal and register on the Mohs scale as a 7. Herkimer Diamond Quartz registers at 7.5 on the Mohs scale. This scale system measures the hardness of a mineral with a diamond rating at a ten.

Quartz crystals can be found in various parts of the world and in a variety of colors: Clear Quartz; Rose Quartz (pink); Amethyst (purple); Citrine Quartz (yellow, golden, orange); Smoky Quartz (gray). Each type contains entirely different properties for healing purposes.

Quartz crystals contain piezoelectric properties. Quartz amplifies, stores, transforms,focuses and transfers energy. Quartz crystals are found in use with: microphones, computers, lasers, ultrasound devices,and also our clocks and wrist watches, to name a few. Quartz crystals are not limited only to physical use, they can also be found in use in metaphysical procedures.

Quartz crystals and gemstones were used by many ancient civilizations, and in recent centuries, by Native American Indians. They are used in many healing ways, as we will explore in more detail throughout this book.

There are a few things to keep in mind pertaining to quartz crystals. They are a consciousness. They have their own energy vibration. This has been proven in many laboratory experiments. Kirlian Photography allows us to view the etheric energies around the crystals. Quartz crystals amplify energy. Thought is a form of energy. Crystals are neutral. They can be used for good or evil. An example is what happened to the lost continent of Atlantis. Use crystals in good health.

MOH'S SCALE

1. Talc (1)
2. Gypsum (2)
3. Calcite (3)
4. Fluorite (4)
5. Apatite (5)
6. Microcline (6)
7. Quartz (7)
8. Topaz (8)
9. Corundum (9) (Ruby and Sapphire)
10. Diamond (10)

Frederick Moh's, a geologist based this scale on the quality of hardness. Hardness in a mineral means the degree of resistance offered by its smooth surface to being scratched. Any mineral in the sequence will be scratched by a harder mineral. Gems are not worthy of cutting and facetting, unless 7 or above.

The Many Types of Quartz

Agate: Banded, Dendritic, Fire, Moss, and Scenic.

Amethyst

Aventurine

Bloodstone

Carnelian

Chalcedony

Chert

Chrysocolla

Chrysoprase

Citrine

Enhydro

Flint

Geode

Jasp-Agate

Jasper: Banded, Poppy, Scenic, or black Touchstone.

Morion (very dark Smoky Quartz)

Novaculite

Onyx

Polyhedroid

Rock Crystal

Rose Quartz

Rutilated Quartz

Sard, Sardonyx

Smoky Quartz

Thunder Egg

Tigereye

The Many Forms of Quartz Crystals

Single Terminated:

Natural quartz crystals come in many sizes, colors and shapes. A quartz crystal has six sides and two ends. The flat end is the base of the crystal that was once rooted into the earth. The other end comes to a point with six facets. This is the terminated end of a crystal. Energy focuses and emanates from this end. These crystals are used by many in meditation and healing practices. Most of the exercises and meditations in this book refer to the use of these particular crystals.

Crystal Clusters:

A crystal cluster is a formation of many single terminated crystals that share a common base. The energy that emanates from this formation is amplified because there are mutiple crystals involved. Crystal clusters are beneficial for placement in a room. They help to raise the vibration of an area. Multiple programming can go into clusters. Also, you can recharge other crystals, gemstones and jewelry by placing them on a crystal cluster. This is done with Clear Quartz or Amethyst clusters, in particular.

Double Terminated:

Double Terminated Crystals are crystals that have a termination point on both ends. These crystals complete a circuit of energy. Energy enters and exits out both ends. They are used by many for healing, meditation, protection and dream work. My favorite Double Terminated Crystal is " Herkimer Diamond " Quartz.

Generator Crystals:

These are large single terminated crystal points. They usually average about five to six inches in length, four inches in diameter, and weigh about one and a half to two and a half pounds. They also come larger. I know a friend who has one that weighs about the same as a cement block, which is twenty five pounds! These crystals are great for using in group meditations and for focusing. They are also nice for meditation altars. Some people place them in a room to alter the environmental vibrations.

Pyramid Facet Crystals:

These are usually Clear Quartz Crystals. A facet may have one or more triangle formations on the surface. These crystals are used for meditations and dream work. There is much information stored inside these crystals. As one sits with a Pyramid Facet Crystal, the knowledge will unfold.

Tabular Crystals:

These are quartz crystals with four narrow sides and two broad sides. Some are found in double terminated form. These are used as " bridgers." They connect us to higher realms. They are used also in Chakra Balancing and are placed in between the chakras.

Crystal Spheres:

These are crystal balls. Energy emanates out of the crystal in <u>all</u> directions. Some people use these for scrying. I use them for meditation. A Rose Quartz sphere is nice to hold during an emotional healing session. Spheres are found in: Clear Quartz, Rutilated Quartz, Amethyst, Rose Quartz, Smoky Quartz, Beryl and others. Clear Quartz is the most common.

Crystal Eggs:

These are oval shaped and are found in many variations similar to the spheres. Crystal eggs are used in healing and meditation. They can be held by a client during a healing session. The practitioner can use them in releasing techniques. Some Polarity Therapists also use them in their session work.

Massage Crystals:

These are Single Terminated crystals that have been polished. The flat base has been rounded off, so it can be held in the hand with more comfort. The terminated end still contains the six facets, but in some cases, the end has been smoothed down. Massage crystals are used in healing practices. The most popular area of use is in body work therapies, such as: Massage, Shiatsu, Polarity Therapy and Reflexology. The crystal point is held over an imbalanced area and gentle pressure is applied. Some people perform " psychic surgery" with these particular crystals.

CRYSTAL BASICS

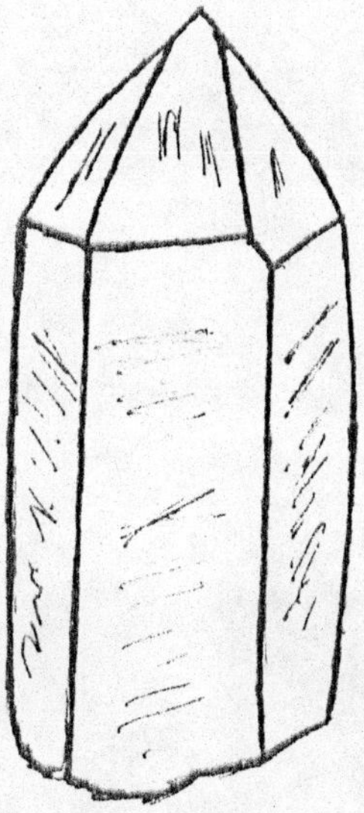

MEETING YOUR CRYSTAL

There are many ways to connect with the world of crystals. You may be given one as a gift, find one on your path during a nature walk, or select one yourself.

Here are some suggestions for choosing a quartz crystal.

SIGHT. You may locate a gem shop in your area and as you look over a group of crystals one or a few seem to catch your eye more than the other ones.

FEEL and SENSE. Once you spot a crystal, pick it up and just see how it feels to you. Quiet your mind and allow the crystal to communicate to you. You have a particular energy vibration and so does each individual crystal. Each one is different and some are more appropriate for you than others.

MUSCLE TEST. You can use Applied Kinesiology, if you and a friend are familiar with this technique. Your friend could "muscle test" you and also you can do her. (For further discussion of this technique, see the chapter on " How to Measure the Energy Centers ".)

PENDULUM. You can use the technique known as, Radiesthesia or " Pendulum Dowsing " to locate a crystal that is appropriate for you. You can also do this for a friend if you want to select one as a gift. All you need is a photograph of them. (If you haven't worked with a pendulum see the article on Dowsing Crystals.)

In reality, the crystal chooses you.

TAKING CARE OF YOUR CRYSTALS

Now that you have your new crystals, you will need to do some basic procedures with them. Quartz crystals are like negative ion generators. They discharge negative ions and collect positive ions. Over a period of time in collecting these positive ions, the crystals begin to loose some of their power. They can become sluggish with the vibrations being less efficient.

It is important to cleanse your crystals so that you can remove these unwanted positive ions. Positive ions can be collected from: microwaves, negative thoughts and feelings, television sets, various other electronic equipment , fluorescent lights, and x-rays at airports. (Have your crystals hand checked.)

Crystals love sunshine. Keep many near your window sills if possible. Also it's good to keep many wrapped for protection. This is very important if you travel and plan to take crystals with you places. I've had too many nice ones get chipped. It's best to wrap them in a natural fabric such as silk or cotton. Whatever color that you wrap them in, the crystal will absorb that color. Some colors that are suggested are: red, violet, blue, gold and white.

You can also keep your crystals in a healing circle pattern. (See the section on charging crystals.) I keep many crystals in my Meditation Room. It's nice to have them handy for holding in meditation. Other crystals are kept near my pillow to aid dreams. Another place that I keep crystals is in my office. This is my Healing Room and it's convenient to have them within reach as I do session work with people for energy balancing. Also many of my clients enjoy holding them during counseling. They aid emotional releasing and help many to feel good about themselves. As you come to use crystals, you will find your own uses and places to keep them.

Cleansing Crystals

- Cover crystals with sea salt for one - three days.

- Salt water Solution: one cup of sea salt to one gallon of distilled or spring water for three to seven days. (For smaller crystals, you can fill a glass up with water and use one teaspoon of sea salt.)

- Bury in the ground for seven days.

- Crystals can be cleansed in ocean water.

- Smudging with sage and cedar. Hold over the smoke of these burning sacred herbs.

- Frankincense can be used for smudging. It is commonly found in the Orient.

- Running mountain stream water for seven days.

- Tears can cleanse crystals (normal saline).

- Crystals can be placed on top of a cleansed Amethyst cluster.

- The element of fire can be used holding the crystals with the terminated end over a candle flame.

- Tibetan tiensha bells can be used. (These are temple bells made from seven different types of metals.)

- Water/ Sun method: Bathe the crystals in distilled or spring water. While the crystals are still wet, place them in direct sunlight for a few days.

For a quick cleansing soak:

Soak the crystals in a solution of sea salt, cider vinegar, and distilled or spring water, completely covered for at least ten minutes or more. The cider vinegar speeds up the action of the salt crystals which absorb the vibrations in the crystals. 1.

a. one cup of sea salt.
b. one cup of cider vinegar.
c. one gallon of spring or distilled water.

Use only as much solution as needed and reserve the unused solution for another time. When you are done cleansing crystals in salt water or sea salt, discard the used portion.

Note: After each therapeutic use of crystals on clients CRYSTALS MUST BE CLEANSED.

1. (Quartz Crystals and Other Gemstones, Crystal Peace, Clyde, N.C. 1984).

My favorite cleansing technique is the salt water solution. This is the most effective and recommended for using on crystals when you first get new ones. The other cleansing I use the most is the salt water /cider vinegar solution. This is a handy formula for quick cleansing baths in between client sessions. For jewelry and some of the other minerals, it is best to cleanse them by covering them in sea salt or smudging them with the sage and cedar. I have found the salt water damaging some of my crystal jewelry. Be careful what you put in the liquids. Quartz by itself does well in the solution baths.

Clearing Crystals

When you first get a crystal, you may want to use it right away. One thing you can do with it is to clear it. When you get a chance later, you can cleanse it more thoroughly. Here are some clearing methods you can use:

THOUGHTS. Energy follows thought. You can mentally clear your crystal by visualizing in your mind's eye that it is being cleared. By adding the affirmation that it is being cleared of any negative energy, this will amplify this process.

BREATH. The power of the breath. Hold a crystal in one hand with your thumb and forefinger holding both ends . Have your other hand hold two opposite sides of the crystal between the thumb and forefinger. Inhale a deep breath and hold it for a moment. As you exhale, squeeze the two sides and visualize the crystal releasing any unwanted energy that it may have accumulated. Blow hard and release that energy from the crystal. Now repeat this again and again, until you have cleared all six sides of the crystal.

As mentioned, the cleansing techniques are better. Your intention is what really counts. Some people combine many of the various clearing and cleansing techniques for some crystals that seem to have accumulated a lot of positive ions and seem lifeless, or don't feel good to hold. For example:

I had a friend who had just received her first crystal for wearing and she wore it out in public one evening. She showed it to a man who was evil in nature. While he held her crystal, he thought negative thoughts about her. He was insecure and jealous concerning her. Later, that night, she had a hard time sleeping. She had nightmares for three nights and felt sick during this time period. She called me up and mentioned what was going on in her life. I told her to immediately come over with the crystal. I held the crystal and began to feel what she had been experiencing. It was necessary to do a few clearing and cleansing techniques. One method alone was not enough to clear the crystal. Each situation is different. You begin to become sensitive as you work with the crystals. This taught a valuable lesson to my friend. Be careful who you let touch your own personal crystals. Their energy also goes into the crystal.

Many times in my healing work, people are drawn to touching my crystals that I may be wearing at the time. I don't get paranoid about it; I just hold the crystal pendant or necklace in my hand and mentally clear it. This is done only when I feel guided to do so, and it is done in a way that is not obvious to anyone else, as not to hurt their feelings. At the end of a day, when I've been doing a few healing sessions, I place my crystal jewelry in sea salt overnight.

There may be times when you do not necessarily want to erase the energy vibration of a crystal. Many crystals are pre-programmed. A perfect example of this are crystals that have pyramid formations / triangles on one or more facets on the terminated end of the crystal. These can be found on some of the Clear Quartz Crystals. Hold the crystal in your hand during a quiet meditation and sense if you receive any information about that particular crystal. If you do need to clear the crystal, you can smudge it and hold the thought that this crystal will continue to contain that memory information.

Another example of not wanting to have a crystal deprogrammed is as follows:

I met a beautiful healer from the Phillipines. He was a psychic surgeon and channeled tremendous power in his healing work. When he was in a trance state doing healing, he channeled the energies of many ascended masters. I wore my crystal during his healing prayers. He blessed it and I didn't want those energies to be erased.

Another example: During my Reiki initiations, I wore a crystal. There is a powerful transference of energy from the Reiki Master to the initiate. The crystal holds the memory of that energy. When I meditate and hold the crystal, I am aware of that spiritual experience.

If you put a crystal into salt water solution or sea salt, it will ERASE the program or memory bank of the crystal.

Remember that when you go through the whole procedure of programming your crystals, which we will discuss later.

Activating and Charging Crystals

Always cleanse crystals before doing these procedures:

- Place crystals in direct sunlight. (The best time is between 11:30 A.M. - 12:30 P.M. and also at sunrise.)
- Place crystals in direct moonlight. (During the winter time you can keep them on a window sill and also hang your crystal pendant with its chain from the window lock. This will catch some moon rays.) Full Moon is best.
- Place crystals inside a pyramid. This will charge the crystals with pyramid energy. (Pyramids are powerful. Try meditating in one!)
- Make a circle with crystals. Place crystals inside the circle. They will become charged in the energy field of the other crystals. Make sure the crystals are pointing into the circle (terminated ends pointing in toward the center of the circle).

Programming Crystals

Quartz crystals store energy. A small quartz chip in a computer holds much data and is its memory bank. On a metaphysical level this realization can also be applied. Here are some suggestions for programming a crystal:

All crystals must be cleansed ahead of time. Crystals can be even more amplified, if they are also charged / activated prior to programming them.

Hold a crystal in your hand. Quiet your mind. Sense what you would like to use this crystal for: healing, meditation, protection, memory recall, for growing things, etc. Once you get a feeling of what you really want to do with that crystal, then project that intention into the quartz crystal. It is that simple. Every time that I give a crystal to a friend as a gift, I cleanse, activate and program it. The program is usually such as this: " May this crystal serve Jane Smith to her highest good. "

If there is something in particular that needs to be programmed, such as a specific desire for healing, here are some other examples:

Colors affect us. Think of the color red. It represents danger and emergency. The traffic light turns red when we are meant to stop. Emergency vehicles all have flashing red lights so others can see them coming and get out of their way. It is a very stimulating color. Red is a good color to use for times of feeling lethargic and sluggish.

If you know of someone who is hyperactive, think of the color blue and program that thought into the crystal. Remember, energy follows thought. There once was a research project done to see the reaction of psychiatric patients in a hospital ward. The ones who had insomnia, slept better with a blue light on in their room.

Green is a healing color for balancing and rejuvenation.

The color orange has been used to balance depression and nervous breakdown.

Yellow stimulates the nerves and is recommended for paralysis and stroke.

Violet is the color vibration of transmutation, as in the Amethyst Quartz crystal.

Pink is the color of universal, unconditional love.

(There are many books on color healing. See the back of this book for listings.)

You can program crystals to help in balancing the chakras. Here is a formula:

Root chakra: RED

Spleen / Navel Chakra: ORANGE

Solar Plexus Chakra: YELLOW

Heart Chakra: GREEN

Throat Chakra: BLUE

Brow Chakra: INDIGO (indigo is a blue / purple).

Crown Chakra: VIOLET

You can select seven cleansed Clear Quartz Crystals to be used for balancing the Major Chakras. They should weigh at least eight ounces each. Purchase or make seven crystal bags that represent the above seven colors. Natural fabrics are best to use for the material. For example: use a RED bag to hold the crystal for balancing the Root Chakra. An ORANGE bag can be used to hold the crystal for balancing the Navel Chakra, etc.

There are many ways to program your chakra crystals. It is suggested to combine a few of these methods:

Use color slides or gels and project the color on the crystal for four to five minutes a day. Project one color at a time for each individual crystal. Do this for at least seven days.

Use music to program the crystal to that particular color vibration. For example:

RED	Key of C	
ORANGE	Key of D	
YELLOW	Key of E	
GREEN	Key of F	
BLUE	Key of G	
INDIGO	Key of A	(indigo is a blue / purple)
VIOLET	Key of B	

You can play a musical instrument on that particular note with a guitar or piano. An easier way, is to play the tape: " Spectrum Suite, " by Steven Halpern. Be sure to get the short version tape. It has music lasting about four minutes in keys: C through B. There is a space of silence in between each key change. Play one note frequency at the same time you are projecting the color onto the crystal. For example: Project the color Red for four to five minutes and at the same time play the key note C. This crystal will be used to balance the Root Chakra located at the base of the spine. If you also visualize along with the music and color, this will amplify the process.

You can program crystals for many other uses:

Garden crystals can be planted in Circle Gardening. The crystal amplifies energy outward to the plants.

Protection crystals: I have a friend who has an interesting occurrence that happens to her. Anytime something major in her life is about to happen to her, her crystal jewelry will fall off. It's like a built in warning system for any crisis.

Crystals can be programmed for specific use in healing.

Meditation crystals can be used for general or specific uses.

Crystals can be programmed to aid you in memory recall. Study for an exam with your crystal, then wear it during the test with the point up.

These are just some suggestions. Let your mind come up with some others for your own personal use.

Another way to program your crystals is to cup your hand around the crystal and breathe the intention into the crystal using the power of the breath. Breathe into the terminated end of the crystal.

Also, some people hold their crystals over the flame of a candle. While they visualize their intention and affirm it, they hold the crystal with the terminated end pointed directly over the flame and rotate it clockwise.

SPIRITUAL MEDICINE CHEST

Below is a list of Crystals & Gemstones that everyone should have for their SPIRITUAL MEDICINE CHEST:

* Smoky Quartz -	grounding energy : good for " spacey ", airy people; transformation crystal : aids those suicidal or addicted to drugs; cleanses the aura.
Apache Tears - (Black Obsidian)	grounding energy; soul reflection (This can be an intense stone for some.)
Pyrite -	grounding energy; increases circulation; digestive aid; strengthens astral body; prosperity manifestation.
* Rose Quartz -	emotional trauma; balances the Heart Chakra; for issues of self-acceptance and unconditonal love.
Rutilated Quartz -	balances chakras, meridians; tissue regeneration; radiation problems; intuitive awakening; balances subtle bodies, especially etheric.
* Clear Quartz -	(It's good to have on hand many sizes and types: single points, clusters, Tabulars, Double Terminated and Generator Crystals.) Amplifies energy; balances the aura; decongests energy blockages; protection; amplifies thoughtforms. Clear Quartz is the <u>only</u> recommended crystal for "through the aura healing ". Master healer.
* "Herkimer Diamond" Quartz -	pain relief; insomnia; energy balancer.
* Tourmalines	(All color varieties)
pink -	emotional healing; balances the Heart Chakra; contains lithium crystals which aid manic depression.
green -	Master healer; balances physical body, nervous system, immune system; opens Heart Chakra.
blue -	spiritual attunement; balances upper chakras.
watermelon -	irregular cellular growth : cancer, pregnancy (developing fetus).
black -	grounding spiritual energy; protection (use with caution.)

* Amber - (a resin)	physical and emotional pain release; cleanses aura; protection .
* Turquoise -	Master healer; Strengthens chakras, meridians, and subtle bodies; stimulates tissue regeneration; aids in increasing circulation; some use it for arthritis.
* Golden and - Madiera Citrine (Quartz)	balances subtle bodies; aids clarity and decision making; aligns lower chakras , especially the Navel and Solar Plexus; raises one's consciousness; a very powerful transition stone : aids suicidals or others who want to grow, but are stubborn about it.
* Aquamarine -	meditative aid; calming; tranquility; reduces inflammation; balances Throat Chakra; etheric body and mental body alignment; headaches; insomnia.
* Lapis Lazuli	meditative aid; activates Throat and Brow Chakras; balances mental body; intuitive awakening; reduces inflammation and infection, especially throat and chest areas; aids dream state.
* Amethyst - (Quartz)	spiritual attunement; activates pineal and pituitary glands, Brow and Crown Chakras; transition stone; spiritual cleansing; alcoholism; headaches; insomnia; protection : can reflect negative energy and also transmute it. (See additonal note at end of this list.)
* Rhodochrosite -	emotional healing : for issues of forgiveness; opens Heart Chakra; nightmares; strengthens : kidneys, pancreas and spleen; integrates the physical, mental, and emotional bodies.

* Kunzite -	emotional healing; balances cardiovascular system; euphoric (contains lithium crystals); alcoholism; manic depression; circulation to extremities; good for massage work. (Leave in area or tape to sore body area.)
* Emerald -	Master balancer; balances Heart Center, meridians and chakras; aligns physical, etheric, emotional bodies; tranquility; harmony; balance; stability; radiation toxicity; attunement to the Universal Life Force and aids alignment of the spine.
* Fluorite -	energy blockages; absorbs, neutralizes and transmutes negative energy; clears a passage for working with crystals and stones in energy balancing work; aids attunement to the Higher Self and the Universe when placed on the upper chakras; mental stimulation and clarity. (I use Fluorite Octahedrons on all of the chakras, in particular, the lower chakras, knees, and feet. I use it with Smoky Quartz at the feet for activating the foot chakras and grounding a person's energy.)
* Topaz -	balances chakras; tension headaches; charges electro-magnetically the physical, emotional and mental bodies and aids creativity; nervous exhaustion; depression; tissue regeneration; balances meridians; joy, playfulness: " allows the child to come out and play ", which is great for workaholics.
Malachite - (Lapis Ligurius)	activates Brow Chakra; stimulates the optic nerve; aids poor eyesight; tissue regeneration; strengthens pineal and pituitary glands; for absorbing and drawing out negative energy in an imbalanced or painful area; meditative aid for soul reflection. Use with caution. This can be a very intense stone!
* Chrysocolla -	arthritis; balances Throat Chakra; calms mind and emotions; strengthens thyroid and lungs; used for breaking up calcifications in one's life.
* Carnelian - (Agate)	digestion aid; grounds energy; stimulates the Second Chakra: procreation; strengthens gallbladder, liver, pancreas; lethargy: increases one's energy output level. (Caution should be applied in using this stone. Hyperactive people somtimes cannot handle the energies of this stone. Be sensitive to each use.)

When I do hospital or house calls, I take a suitcase of crystals and gemstones with me. I meditate ahead of time and I am guided to take along certain ones for particular issues. The ones marked with an asterisk * usually come on all calls.

When you transport your crystals and minerals, it is suggested to have each one individually wrapped. You can use a large section of material to wrap many crystals. Just roll a section and cover a crystal, then roll another section and cover a crystal, etc. Again, it is important to use natural fiber material. Many practitioners use cotton that has been dyed red. Red cloth protects crystals from taking on any other energies, than that of the crystals. Think about it. It is important if you have many crystals with their own individual programming. You may not want to mix them all up together. Also the energy in some institutions can be overwhelming and draining.

As you begin to become acquainted with the qualities and properties of each crystal and gemstone, you will come to know your own sensitivity in working with them. It is the minerals who are the true teachers of the mineral kingdom. As you join your forces together in service to humanity and the universe, you will overcome limitations. New doors and new worlds will open up for you. Go and serve others. It's why you are really here.

A final note on the listing of the crystals. I had mentioned more discussion on Amethyst. Some hyperactive people are not compatible with this particular quartz. I knew a woman who purchased an Amethyst for her young daughter once. Soon as they got it, they cleansed it. When it came time to dry the crystal, they placed it on a towel. They later came back for it and the crystal had disappeared! The woman called to tell me of her story and I asked her if her daughter was by any chance, hyperactive. She said she was. If you are not meant to have a particular crystal, you won't.

Another interesting Amethyst story I want to share was told to me, by a friend, Ginny. She was having a birthday party for her child and had invited many children and their parents and some of her relatives over. Ginny thought it would be nice to place an Amethyst Quartz cluster in the room where everyone would be for the whole day. She also felt guided to wear a pendant for protection, since she felt that some of the people who were to come were negative in nature. When the party was over and everyone had left, Ginny went over to collect her Amethyst cluster. She noticed that it had completely lost all of its color! I had sold the quartz to her and remembered that it had been a dark Amethyst. This is just an example of the fact that the mineral kingdom is working for us whether we are aware of it, or not. Ginny and I both felt that the crystal had transmuted a lot of the negative vibrations that these people may have been carrying around with them. I suggested that she cleanse the cluster in sea salt water for seven days and then plant the quartz in the ground.

My intention for writing this book was not to get into lengthy descriptions on the properties of quartz crystals and various gemstones. This book is about application techniques for meditation and healing. If you are interested in more information on the metaphysical properties of minerals, then I suggest that you read the following books and also the ones listed at the back of this book.

Gem Elixirs and Vibrational Healing, Vol. 1 by Gurudas.

Healing Stoned by Lorusso & Glick.

Spiritual Value of Gemstones by Richardson & Huett.

Crystal Enlightenment by Raphaell.

HERKIMER STORIES

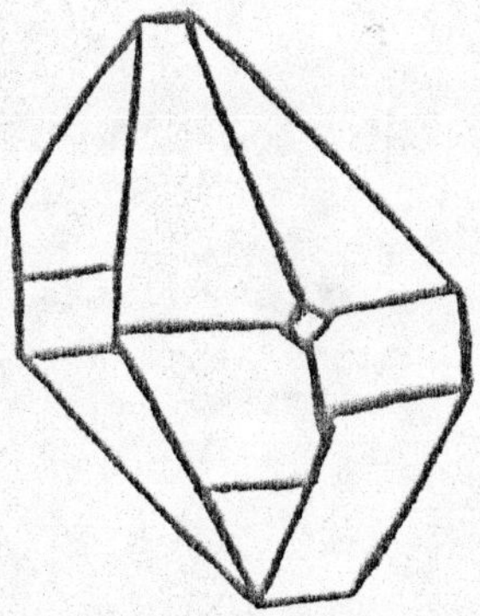

Pain = Energy Blockage / Congestion of Energy

The greater the pain, the greater the energy blockage.

Herkimers are very, special crystals. They are Double Terminated Crystals, known as " Herkimer Diamonds ". They are usually found in Clear Quartz, but I have seen a few in Smoky Quartz color. Herkimers can be found in upper state New York, in Herkimer County. They are my favorite Double Terminated Crystals.

Herkimers are used for:

- Vision Quests.
- Dream Work.
- In and Out of Body Experiences (Astral Travel).
- Healing Work for releasing physical pain.

Vision Quest is a way of soul searching. There are preliminary acts that one may do in preparing for this event. Some Native Americans do a Sweat Lodge Ceremony of Purification prior to going on a Vision Quest. They then go out into nature for at least three days and nights with some water. They eat no food and some do not sleep. Alone with nature in a prayerful, meditative state, they bring themselves into alignment with their Higher Self and the Universe. Some see visions and some are given a new name to that vision.

Herkimers aid this spiritual experience tremendously. I once asked a Native American crystal teacher, Oh Shinnah, if she ever used Herkimers on a vision quest before. She shared that at one time she went on a quest for over twenty one days and had taken a Herkimer crystal with her. It had been a very powerful experience for her.

Herkimers are great for those who are having some difficulty in sleeping. They are a conscious tool for dreamwork. Herkimers are used for out of body experiences. (When we sleep at night, our astral body leaves us to journey onto another plane.) If you find yourself with insomnia some night, then try the exercise on the following page.

Find and obtain a Herkimer crystal. Lie down with your Herkimer. Do the Relaxation Breath Technique. (You'll find a description of this method on page 33.) Hold the Herkimer in your LEFT hand. If it is small, then just place it in your palm center and keep your hand open and relaxed.

Do a " Body Check " starting with your feet. Ask yourself, " Is my left foot tense or relaxed ? " (pause.) " Is my left calf tense or relaxed ? " (pause.) " Is my left knee tense or relaxed ? " (pause.) " Is my left thigh tense or relaxed ? " (pause.) " Is my left hip tense or relaxed ? " (pause.) Then go to your right side and repeat the body check. If you come to an area that is tense just acknowledge that it is so and go on to another area. You begin the Body Check Technique with the feet and continue up to the head.

By the time you have gone over each body section from feet to head (about five to ten minutes), you should be very relaxed. The Herkimer crystal adds to your relaxation as you hold it.

Herkimers are great for dreamwork. I keep a pad and pen by my bed each night, so when I awaken in the morning I can recall my dreams. If you do this first thing in the morning, it will help you to remember your dreams. Sometimes I even keep a tape recorder near by. I did this once and repeated my dream into the recorder and was able to write a story from it. Haven't you ever had a dream that was so fantastic that you thought even Hollywood could make a movie out of it ?

Many messages come to us in our dreams. Any crystal will enhance your dream state and Herkimers are one of the best ! It helps if you program your crystal for dream recall. Every night affirm to yourself that you will remember your dreams. You can purchase or make a bag to hold your crystal in at night. It should be made out of a natural fabric such as silk or cotton. The bag can be a small one for wearing (with a neck string), or a larger one that fits in your pillow case. As long as the crystal is in your energy field, it will continue to affect you. I have a bookcase at the top of my bed. This allows me room to have several crystals, plus I also wear different ones for my dreams.

It's also good to read your notes on your dream and take that information into a conscious, meditative state. Many things begin to surface into our awareness when this is done.

Herkimers help to release physical pain. One night I had the flu - body ache, no energy, especially my back area. I ached so much that I couldn't sleep. I placed a palm size Herkimer under my back on one side along the spine. My lower back really was hurting. I kept the crystal there for three to five minutes then I moved it to another aching area. I continued to repeat this until one side felt completed. Next I placed the Herkimer at my lower back on the other side for three to five minutes. Then the crystal was moved up to another imbalanced area. On completion of both sides, my strength came back, the pain subsided or was completely gone and I slept like a baby. (I should mention that I sleep on a water bed. If you find sleeping on " rocks " uncomfortable, then just use a smaller size.)

Pregnancy is another situation that calls for Herkimers. They aid lower back pain and they can also be held in one or both hands during labor contractions. Good Luck !

A word of caution is necessary when using Herkimer crystals. Most people cannot wear Herkimers. They have a tendency to " space " people out. If you are a very grounded person then this may not be an issue for you. I have seen some people that were " spacey." (Their heads are " up in the clouds " so to speak.) They would try to wear " Herks " and they would walk around lightheaded and not be totally aware of what they were doing. Herkimers are for meditation and dreamwork. Be aware .

MEDITATING WITH CRYSTALS

HOW TO USE THIS BOOK

Read through each of the healing meditations and exercises. It's good to do this at least twice, especially for the lengthy ones. First, you'll get a basic idea of how it all goes. The second time, you can break each segment down. It will help you to gather up your supplies of what is needed and get a sense when to introduce each crystal into the experience.

These procedures are especially helpful if a friend reads them as you practice the exercises. It works well also should a teacher choose to share some of these healing meditations or techniques with his / her class.

Keep in touch with your sensations during each exercise. Take mental notes of your experiences and on completion write down what occurred. There are blank pages after some of the exercises for your own note taking.

Before doing any of the following meditations and exercises, it is important to become in tune with one's self. I am including two exercises that will assist one to become attuned to his / her self more easily:

First, there is the RELAXATION BREATH exercise:

Get in a comfortable position. This can be a Yoga semi-lotus on the floor, sitting in a chair, or lying down. What ever feels good for you. Close your eyes and take some slow, deep breaths. Inhale through your nostrils and exhale out through your mouth. Each time that you INHALE, visualize the word, RELAXATION. You are inhaling relaxation each time you breathe in through your nostrils. Each time you EXHALE through your mouth allow your body and mind to exhale away all tension. Release tension each time you exhale. Let go of all stress. Inhale relaxation and exhale away all tension. Just let it go now....

Pause for about four minutes.

OUR MANY SELVES

Subconscious	-	Child within	-	Lower Self
Conscious	-	Adult	-	Middle Self
Superconscious	-	Parent	-	Higher Self

The second exercise is the SOUL ATTUNEMENT exercise. The following is a brief version. We have three levels of mind:
conscious = Adult; subconscious = Child; and superconscious = Parent.

It is important to connect with all three levels for meditation and healing work.

SOUL ATTUNEMENT (brief version)

Get in a relaxed postion. Do the Relaxation Breath exercise. Begin to relax and deepen.....

" There are many parts of your being that make you whole. Call on the child within you to come out and play. " (Pause.) The child has surfaced. (Pause.) Now, see the child playing in front of you.
Pause for about two minutes.

Now, call on the adult part of your being and allow it to surface and come out and play. Pause for one minute. Now, see the adult surfaced and playing. (Pause.) See the adult playing with the child. They are together as one. Pause for two minutes.

Now, call on the parent within your being and allow that part of yourself to surface. (Pause.) The parent has surfaced and is now present in front of you. Allow the parent to play with the child and the adult. All are playing child, adult and parent...the child, adult and parent of your being. See all three playing in a circle...all three as one unit... one circle. Pause for two to three minutes. Notice how you feel inside as you witness all these aspects of your being. Compare this with how you felt before you began this exercise.

Everyone responds differently to this exercise. The more you practice this, the easier it will come to you. It will also give you a clear view of any issues that you may have hidden. They will come to the surface for you to look at and work through. Most people begin doing this exercise three times a day the first week. Then the second week, it is done twice a day. Then eventually, it is done once a day. It is a perfect way to begin each day. This exercise puts you in attunement with all three levels of your being. After some practice of this technique, you'll be able to attune to all three levels instantly upon willing it. I call this technique, the " Soul Attunement " because it helps you to sense a clearer connection with your Higher Self. When I have shared it with others, it has been a very powerful experience for some.

MY PERSONAL EXPERIENCE:

GROUNDING YOURSELF

Visualize growing luminous roots down through your feet into the floor and then into the earth. See your roots continue to grow deeper into the earth.

Another way to do this is to hold any of the grounding stones in your left hand. You also could place them at your feet instead. Again visualize growing luminous roots through your feet. You are directing your energy downward into the earth. The grounding stones will assist this process.

As you become more sensitive to working with energy, then you will feel the difference of grounding your energy with and without the grounding stones.

GROUNDING STONES

First choice: Smoky Quartz and Black Tourmaline

Second choice: Apache Tears

Third choice: Pyrite

Fourth choice: Agates

I find the Apache Tears denser than the Smoky Quartz in grounding energy. The Apache Tears (black obsidian) are an intense grounding stone. Be sensitive when working with this one.

HEALING CHANNEL MEDITATION

This meditation can be done with one or two people. If two people are doing this exercise, one will stand behind a person who is seated.

Relax and center yourself. Once you are relaxed and centered you can connect your hands to the shoulders of the person in front of you. (If you are doing this on yourself, place your hands where you want to direct healing energy.)

Visualize a beam of light above your head. This light represents healing energy coming down from the Heavens. Allow healing energy to enter into your Crown Chakra at the top of your head. As you take that energy in, direct it down to your heart.

Breathe in the Healing Love Light of the Universe... the Divine Essence... the Prana...the Life force. Take this Healing Light Energy into your Crown Chakra and see it going down into your Heart Chakra. It is your birthright to receive this healing energy. Pause one to two minutes.

See your heart center, your Heart Chakra being filled up with healing energy. You are filling up your heart with an unlimited supply of healing energy. Continue to breathe in the Healing Love Light of the Universe.

See and feel your heart expanding, Sense it stretching and growing as you continue to fill up your heart with the Healing Love Light. Pause two minutes.

Visualize two beams of healing light coming out of the top of your heart. One light ray goes to the right and the other goes to the left. See the healing light energies going to the top of your shoulders, then down your arms and to your hands. Focus on the healing energy and direct it out through your hands.

Direct the healing energy out of your hands and onto the shoulders of the person in front of you. Be aware of how warm your hands get.

You are the instrument, the vehicle for channeling the Healing Love Light of the Universe. Continue to fill your vessel with this healing energy.

The more you are receptive to receiving this healing energy, the more you will channel. The supply is unlimited.

When you are finished channeling healing energy to your friend, trade places. Its that simple. The more you practice this, the better you'll get at it. It is a gift we are all born with. Some just know how to use it better.

HEALING CHANNEL MEDITATION

This meditation can be done with one or two people. If two people are doing this exercise, one will stand behind a person who is seated.

Relax and center yourself. Once you are relaxed and centered you can connect your hands to the shoulders of the person in front of you. (If you are doing this on yourself, place your hands where you want to direct healing energy.)

Visualize a beam of light above your head. This light represents healing energy coming down from the Heavens. Allow healing energy to enter into your Crown Chakra at the top of your head. As you take that energy in, direct it down to your heart.

Breathe in the Healing Love Light of the Universe... the Divine Essence... the Prana...the Life force. Take this Healing Light Energy into your Crown Chakra and see it going down into your Heart Chakra. It is your birthright to receive this healing energy. Pause one to two minutes.

See your heart center, your Heart Chakra being filled up with healing energy. You are filling up your heart with an unlimited supply of healing energy. Continue to breathe in the Healing Love Light of the Universe.

See and feel your heart expanding, Sense it stretching and growing as you continue to fill up your heart with the Healing Love Light. Pause two minutes.

Visualize two beams of healing light coming out of the top of your heart. One light ray goes to the right and the other goes to the left. See the healing light energies going to the top of your shoulders, then down your arms and to your hands. Focus on the healing energy and direct it out through your hands.

Direct the healing energy out of your hands and onto the shoulders of the person in front of you. Be aware of how warm your hands get.

You are the instrument, the vehicle for channeling the Healing Love Light of the Universe. Continue to fill your vessel with this healing energy.

The more you are receptive to receiving this healing energy, the more you will channel. The supply is unlimited.

When you are finished channeling healing energy to your friend, trade places. Its that simple. The more you practice this, the better you'll get at it. It is a gift we are all born with. Some just know how to use it better.

MY PERSONAL EXPERIENCE:

CRYSTAL MANIFESTATION MEDITATION

Supplies needed:

One Clear Quartz Crystal

Paper and a pen / pencil

Relax and center yourself. Sit in silence for five minutes.
Pause for five minutes.

Draw or write your request on paper. This can be a drawing or an affirmation.

Fold the paper three or four times until it is palm size.

Hold the crystal in your LEFT hand with the point inward towards the shoulder. At the same time, hold the paper with the request in your RIGHT hand. As you hold these for five minutes, remain in a neutral, receptive mode. Be open to receive without attachment.

Place the paper in the LEFT hand. Place the crystal in the RIGHT hand with the crystal point directed out away from the body. This is the sending mode. Send your request out to the Universe. You may say, " This crystal is to assist me with my intention and to serve me to my highest good." Pause for five minutes. Again, remain neutral. Make this goal or desire a preference, not an attachment.

While holding the paper and crystal in each hand, bring both hands together. Hold them at your chest area for about three minutes. You may finish with the saying, " It is good. It is done. So be it."

MY PERSONAL EXPERIENCE:

CRYSTAL HEALING MEDITATION

Time: ± 25 minutes

Supplies: one Clear Quartz Crystal (at least 3 oz. in weight)

(Note: This exercise is not recommended for people wearing heart pacemakers.)

Get in a relaxed position. Do the Soul Attunement to help center yourself.

- Hold the crystal in BOTH hands and go into a prayerful, meditative state.

- Sense the emotion of love and project love into the crystal.

- Project your favorite color into the crystal.

- Lie down with your back against a flat surface.

- Place the crystal over the Heart Chakra area and continue being in a relaxed meditative state.

- Visualize a heart inside the crystal.

- See the heart begin to expand and grow.

- See the heart become larger and larger.

- See the heart inside the crystal becoming warmer as it becomes larger.

- See the heart expanding so much that it completely fills the crystal.

- The heart is so big now that it begins to push against the walls of the crystal.

- It stretches so much that it bursts out of the crystal and continues to grow.

- It expands across your heart and chest sending healing love all over your body. Bathe in this healing love light. Know that it is your birthright to receive this healing love. You are worthy to receive this love. Love yourself so that you can go and love others.

- When you feel completed, sit up again and sense how you feel.

MY PERSONAL EXPERIENCE:

SENSITIVITY EXERCISE with MALACHITE

You will need one Malachite stone.

Sit in a comfortable position. Place a Malachite in both of your hands. Do the Relaxation Breath and allow yourself to relax and center. Be in this quiet space for five to ten minutes. Pause.

Place the Malachite in your LEFT hand. Take your RIGHT hand and stretch it out in front of you. Close your eyes and slowly direct your right hand (with open palm) towards your forehead area. Malachite activates the Brow Chakra. Sense how close your hand needs to be in front of your forehead area; before you sense pressure between your hand and your forehead. After you have measured this distance pause for a moment and sense how you feel.

Put down the Malachite stone and rub your hands together briskly for about two minutes. This activates the palm chakras in your hand.

Again close your eyes and stretch your RIGHT hand out in front of you. Bring your RIGHT hand (open palm) towards your forehead area. Sense if there is any difference in how close your hand came to sensing your Brow Chakra. Your sensitivity this time should have doubled !

MY PERSONAL EXPERIENCE:

GROUP CRYSTAL MEDITATIONS

Meditation # 1:

Form a circle holding hands. Sit in a comfortable position. Quiet your mind. Do the Relaxation Breath. Pause for two minutes. Close your eyes and visualize a very large Clear Quartz Crystal above the center of the group. See the large crystal coming down from the Heavens. The point of the crystal is aimed downward at the center of the circle. See luminous cords descending down from the crystal point into the center of the circle. Each cord is a different hue and color. Feel yourself connecting with the different colored cords. The etheric cords weave in and out and around the circle. They blend the energies of each person and combine these energies as one. Pause for five to ten minutes.

Meditation # 2:

Place a large Generator Crystal in the center of a room. Form a circle holding hands. Sit in a comfortable postion. Quiet the mind and do the Relaxation Breath. Pause two minutes. Focus your attention on the <u>center</u> crystal. Visualize a beam of healing light coming out of the crystal and aiming in your direction. It is aimed at your Heart Center. Allow your heart to receive this healing light ray. Allow you heart to grow and expand. Pause for ten minutes.

Meditation # 3: Planetary Earth Healing

Supplies: One globe of the Planet Earth.

One crystal for each person.

Each person invoved in this group meditation needs to bring one personal crystal to this exercise. Finger or palm size Clear Quartz Crystals will do. Place a globe of the Planet Earth in the center of a room. Have each person place his or her personal crystal beside the globe. The crystals need to be pointed in toward the globe. The crystals form a circle around the globe with the crystal points aimed toward the globe. Form a circle holding hands. (It is important that each person be in direct line with the personal crystal that he or she placed next to the globe. If you have a very large group, this might not be possible to do.) Sit in a comfortable position. Quiet your mind. Do the Relaxation Breath. Do the Healing Channel Meditation. Pause for four minutes.

Focus on a beam of healing energy pouring out of your heart area. Direct this healing light into the center of the circle. See the circle of crystals that surrounds the globe connecting their energies. As the crystals amplify the energy of the group they are reinforced with their circle pattern. See the crystal energy begin to spiral upward and revolve around the globe in a clockwise motion. This is our mother, Mother Earth. Send healing love and support to Mother Earth. Direct this healing energy to all of her troubled areas and to all her troubled peoples. Pause for five minutes. Visualize a golden ray completely surrounding the planet Earth. It is like an etheric band-aid. It covers and heals all of her wounds. Continue to send healing light until the group feels completed.

BATHING WITH CRYSTALS

One day I was selling crystals at a Psychic Fair. A lady came up to me and inquired about the use of quartz crystals in taking a shower. I suspected her source of interest and asked if she had read Shirley MacLaine's book, " Dancing in the Light " . She had read it, also. In Shirley's book she briefly mentions that when she takes a shower each day, she uses four quartz crystals. She mentions nothing else in reference to how she uses them, nor are crystals mentioned anywhere else in the book. I decided to explore this one further. I meditated with crystals and came up with the following techniques. I thank Shirley MacLaine for this inspiration. Share these bath exercises with your friends. You'll convert shower traditionalists to bath addicts.

Gather the following supplies, then read through the exercises two times before doing the baths. Some of the exercises are lengthier than others because there are more details and steps to follow. Begin with a Basic Crystal Bath first; then approach the more advanced ones. These baths will balance your chakras and energy; relax you physically, mentally and emotionally; energize and renew you. You'll wonder why you waited so long to getting around to doing them. If you are into baths more than showers, you'll never go back to your old bathing pattern.

Always take a shower or a bath prior to the Crystal Baths. The Crystal Baths are for spiritual cleansing. It is important to be cleansed ahead of time.

Basic Crystal Bath

Supplies needed:

apple cider vinegar

sea salt

measuring cup

Also Needed

sage and cedar herbs for smudging

abalone sea shell or a burning dish for herbs

one feather of a bird: crow. hawk, turkey, etc. The larger, the better.

** cassette player (no Walkmans in the tub!)

music tapes: Classical or New Age Music

incense (optional)

candles

matches

1 large Fluorite Octahedron (palm size)

2 palm size Clear Quartz Crystals

2 palm size Amethyst Quartz crystals. (If you are hyperactive in nature, then replace the Amethyst points with Clear Quartz single point crystals.)

Draw your bath water. Measure and pour in one cup of Cider vinegar and one cup of sea salt. Place quartz crystals and Fluorite along side of the tub for later use. Light candles and incense. Get the tape player ready to play your music. (You can turn it on right before you get into the tub. This way, the music will last longer and you won't have to disturb your bath to get out and turn it over.) Once your bath is filled to the level that you want, then it is time to burn the sacred herbs. Fill the abalone shell or burning dish with sage and cedar and light the herbs. Be sure to open a window or door to the outside, so that any negative energy that may be released goes outside.

** Please note: Make sure that your cassette player is away from the tub area. Be careful in touching it. There's always a chance of it short circuiting from the steam or wet hands.

Once you have lit the herbs, use the feather to fan the smoke. Go over to the tub and smudge your bathing space. Next smudge the whole bath room. Lastly, smudge yourself front and back. (You can use the feather to fan the smoke in front of your body and to the sides.) Some people like to cup the smoke in their hands and direct it over specific places of the body. You can hold the shell behind your back and direct the smoke to go where you want it to.

Do a Soul Attunement on yourself to center your energy. Pause a minute. If you want, you can bless the bath water. Here's a sample blessing;

" May this cleansing bath cleanse my being on all levels: spiritually, mentally, emotionally, etherically and physically. May this healing bath serve me to the highest good. "

Turn on the relaxation music. Turn off or dim the lights. Get in the tub. Immerse yourself completely three times. Pause a minute. Take the crystals and Fluorite and place them in the tub. Put the large Fluorite at the bottom of the tub BETWEEN both feet. Take one Clear Quartz and place it on the outside of your LEFT foot with the point going towards your shoulder. Take an Amethyst crystal and place it on the outside of your RIGHT foot. Point the Amethyst away from your body. Take the remaining two crystals and hold one in each hand. The LEFT hand can hold the Clear Quartz with the point going towards the shoulder. The RIGHT hand can hold the Amethyst crystal with the point going away from the body.

Do the Relaxation Breath holding the crystals in your hands and also be aware of the ones at your feet. Breathe in relaxation. Exhale and release all tension and stress. Allow yourself to relax and let go. Pause a few minutes.

Visualize healing energy entering the LEFT side of your body. See it healing and rejuvenating you as it travels up and around your body. The energy exits out your RIGHT side. It takes away any tension, stress, or blockages that may have been held there. As you let go of any imbalances in your body, you will fill those areas with the healing light energy. Bathe in this healing light and enjoy the music. Allow all of your senses to be activated. You feel the comfort of the bathing water, smell the incense, and hear the soothing music filling you on many levels. Be at peace with yourself. Allow yourself to be renewed. Continue bathing until you feel completed. When you are done, be sure to cleanse the used crystals in a saltwater solution for a few days.

MY PERSONAL EXPERIENCE:

Recommended Audio Tapes for Crystal Baths

	Title	Artist
	Harmonic Choir, Vol. I	David Hykes
	Spectrum Suite (extended version)	Steven Halpern
*	Name Divine Series: (chants, nature sounds, very powerful) comes in the following traditions: Christian, Judaic, Islamic, Vedic and Buddhist.	Brother Charles
*	Inside the Great Pyramid	Paul Horn
	Natural Light	Halpern/Smith
*	A Rainbow Path	Kay Gardner
	Aura Sound: Vols. I or II	William Aura
	Golden Voyage: Vols. I, II, III, or IV	Dexter
	Silk Road	Kitaro
*	Down to the Moon Caverna Magica	Vollenweider
	Tibetan Bells	Wolff
*	Divine Gypsy	Yogananda
	Essence Violet Joy	Joel Andrews
	Ancient Echoes	Halpern/Kelly
	Snowflakes Are Dancing	Tomita/Isao

These are only a few suggestions for music to drift away on. I've marked my favorites with an asterisk. For more music listings, write for our Music Catalog.

CRYSTAL CLEANSING BATH

Use the same supplies and do the same preparations as the Basic Crystal Bath with the following additions:

You'll need two sets of four finger size Clear Quartz Crystals. (Place these next to the bath tub.)

You may have a vibrational essence that you would like to add at a later use. (This is optional.) Keep the bottle outside along the tub. Some suggestions: Amethyst elixir or Crab Apple flower remedy.

Once you have made all of the bath preparations do the following:

Take one set of the Clear Quartz Crystals into your hands. Program these crystals to aid you in releasing your emotions into it for later purposes. Place a crystal in each corner of the bath tub. Make sure the terminated end with the point is facing out away from the tub water.

Before entering the bath water, clear the area by drawing a counter-clockwise circle three times over the water with your hand. You may add a prayer if you feel guided to do so.

Enter the water and immerse yourself at least one time. Get into a relaxed state by doing the Relaxation Breath. Once you are relaxed and centered, get in touch with your emotions. This is a perfect setting for letting go of any issues that you need to release. The crystals in each corner are in the proper position for releasing. By having the points away from you, you are able to put into the crystals any unwanted energies. They will collect and store those energies.

Release into each crystal, one at a time, all unwanted emotions, thoughts and feelings. Exhale anger, releasing it into the crystal. When you have finished releasing anger, move on to another crystal and release another emotion into it. Whatever your issues are at the moment, continue to work on releasing them. Some emotions to release are: frustration, resentment, hatred, anxiety, jealousy and envy, to name a few. One by one, release into each crystal until you have released all negativities and have completed your efforts. When you feel complete with the releasing, take the crystals out of each corner. Place them outside next to the tub.

Now take the other unused set of four crystals and place them in each corner of the tub. This time the points will be aimed at the center of the tub toward you. These are for directing healing energies from the Universe to you. Visualize bathing in healing light. Be aware that these crystals are amplifying your energy field with healing light.

You may add a vibrational essence at this time. Bathe in the balancing water and feel the vibrations of the essence renewing you.

Continue bathing until you feel completed.

When you are finished, soak the used crystals in a salt water solution for cleansing.

MY PERSONAL EXPERIENCE:

CHAKRA BALANCING - CRYSTAL BATHING EXERCISE

Measure your Energy Centers. (See the chapter on chakras for details.)

Gather the same supplies as in the Basic Crystal Bath with the following exception: replace the Amethyst crystals with Clear Quartz Crystals.

Also gather two sets of four finger size crystals. These will be placed in the tub corners as described in the Crystal Cleansing Bath.

Do the same preparations as stated in the Basic Crystal Bath exercise. Also put the first set of finger crystals in each tub corner. The first set will have the crystal points facing away from the center.

Enter the water and immerse yourself three times. Get into a relaxed state. Pause for a few minutes. Focus on each corner crystal. Release into each crystal any unwanted emotion or thought. Pause for five minutes. After you have completed releasing into the crystals, remove them away from the tub.

Place the unused set of finger crystals into each tub corner. This time the points will be aimed into the center of the tub toward you. The crystals will amplify your balancing work.

Place two palm size crystals at your feet and two in your hands. Crystals on the LEFT side of the body are pointed toward your shoulder. Crystals on the RIGHT side of the body are pointed away from you shoulder.

Do the Relaxation Breath. Pause for three minutes.

Place the LEFT hand with the crystal over your HEART center. Place the RIGHT hand with the crystal over the SOLAR PLEXUS area. Have the crystals in both hands poining up toward your head. Pause for three minutes. Be aware of what is happening to your energy.

Take the LEFT hand and place it over your THROAT area. Have the crystal pointing up towards your head. Take the RIGHT hand and place it below the NAVEL area with the point aimed up towards the shoulders. Pause for three minutes.

Take the LEFT hand with the crystal and hold it over the BROW center. The crystal should be pointed up towards the top of the head. Take the RIGHT hand with the crystal and place it over the GENITALS area. Again have the crystal point aimed up towards the shoulders. (An alternative to this position is to turn on your left side and hold the right hand over the COCCYX area, at the base of the spine.) Pause for three minutes.

After the six chakra areas have been balanced, take the LEFT hand and place it over the CROWN of the head. The crystal point should be aimed at the front of the body. Visualize healing light balancing the Crown Chakra. Take the RIGHT hand and place it over the HEART center with the crystal point aimed up. A right hand alternative could be to just rest it along your right side. Pause for three minutes.

Take your RIGHT hand and rest it along your right side. Take the LEFT hand and point the crystal at the top of your head. Next draw a line with the crystal point from the CROWN center to the BROW center. Continue to connect the energies by drawing a line from the BROW center to the THROAT center. Next, continue drawing a line from the THROAT center to the HEART center, then the HEART to the SOLAR PLEXUS, then the SOLAR PLEXUS to below the NAVEL area and finally from the NAVEL area to the GENITALS area. Visualize closing your chakras for protection.

Remove the crystals from your hands and brush down your energy field. Do this a few times, while gently stroking your aura and body downward from head to feet.

Hold your feet and grow luminous roots . Ground your energy by visualizing your energy going down deep into Mother Earth. Pause for two minutes. This is important to do. I find that this crystal exercise can sometimes make you lightheaded and grounding your energy helps.

MY PERSONAL EXPERIENCE:

Bathing with Crystals for Spiritual Cleansing

Use a Quartz Crystal Pendulum and measure the energy of your chakras. Check to see which way the pendulum rotates: clockwise vs. counter clockwise. Most readings will reveal counter clockwise before doing any of these balancing exercises.

Cleanse your body by taking a shower or bath to remove dirt, oils,etc.

Smudge environment and bath space.

Draw a bath. Fill the tub full and add:
- 1 cup of apple cider vinegar
- 1 cup of sea salt.

Set up a healing environment: a quiet house. (Send your children, if you have any,to the neighbors so you won't be disturbed.)
- quiet space
- incense (optional)
- candles or dim light
- relaxing music
- crystals, as described in the Basic Crystal Bath with the addition of two sets of four finger size crystals. (One set is for releasing and the other set is for after the discharge.)
- Sa die Balancing Oil or another type of anointing oil. (optional)

Take set # 1 of the four finger crystals and place one crystal in each of the four corners of the tub. The crystals should be pointing out away from the center of the tub. Place all of the other crystals and special oil next to the tub. This way they'll be within reach for later use.

Now, you are ready to begin. Lights dimmed...music playing...go for it! Before entering into the tub, say a prayer over the water. You can also use the Crystal Pendulum by rotating it clockwise (in a positive motion) over the water.

Prayer suggestion: "Father, Mother, Son as One: I pray that this cleansing bath will cleanse and renew my being on all levels. This cleansing water is filled with the Healing Light of the Universe. As I cleanse my being on all levels, I will be rejuvenated and renewed."

When you are ready, enter into the Cleansing Bath. Immerse yourself fully (head too) three times.

Take the large crystals that you placed on the floor outside the tub. Place as follows:

Large Fluorite Octahedron between both feet.

Large Clear Quartz at the LEFT foot (on the outside) and also one in the LEFT hand with the crystals pointing up toward the upper body.

Place an Amethyst crystal at the RIGHT foot (on the outside) and also one in the RIGHT hand. The points should be aimed away from the upper body. (You can replace the Amethyst with other large Clear Quartz, if you are a hyperactive person.) Now, settle in for a few moments getting relaxed. Pause for four minutes.

When you are ready, focus on the small crystals that you placed in each tub corner with the points facing <u>out</u>. You will continue holding the large palm crystals and the other large crystals are at your feet.

RELEASING TECHNIQUE

Focus your attention on each of the four corner crystals that have their points <u>out</u>. Breathe in the Relaxation Breath and breathe out all tension and stress. Direct your attention into the front LEFT corner crystal. Release your tension and your stress into that crystal. Energy follows thought. Direct your releasing into the left front crystal. As you exhale away tension (or a particular emotion) direct it into the left crystal; do this nine times. Nine is the number of forgiveness. Release into the left crystal nine times. (Pause.)

Now focus on the front RIGHT corner crystal. Breathe in relaxation and exhale away tension and stress. Release any unwanted thoughts or feelings into the right crystal. Release into the crystal nine times. (Pause.)

Next, focus on the rear crystal behind you on your right. Release and discharge into this crystal nine times. (Pause.)

Lastly, focus on the rear crystal behind you on your left side. Release into it nine times. Remember that on your last few releases to really let go. Breathe out all unwanted thoughts and feelings. (Pause.)

You now have completed the releasing / discharging part of this cleansing bath. Now, drain the tub half way. Take the four corner crystals and remove them away from the tub.

You should still have a second set of small crystals. Take these four crystals and place them in each corner of the tub. This time the crystal points will be pointed inward toward the center of the tub.

Fill the remainder of the tub with warm water. (If you can stand hot water, then that will help to relax you more. Be careful of very hot tubs if you are in advanced stages of a pregnancy.) At this time you could add the Sá die Balancing Oil, another oil, or flower / crystal essence remedy. Add a few drops.

Immerse yourself fully one time.

Become relaxed and settled in your bath again. Hold the palm crystals as before and have the other large ones near your feet.

Visualize a connection with your new set of corner crystals. Energy follows thought. Connect with the FRONT LEFT corner crystal (#1). Visualize a golden ray of light coming out of the crystal. Take that golden ray and connect it with the FRONT RIGHT corner crystal (# 2). Once the energies of the crystals are connected, visualize the golden ray coming out of the (#2) crystal and connecting with the RIGHT REAR corner crystal (#3). Again, visualize the golden ray coming out of the (#3) crystal and connecting with the remainder LEFT REAR corner crystal (#4). Connect that crystal (#4) back to the first crystal in the FRONT LEFT corner (#1). You now have completed the crystal connection into a square pattern.

You now can strengthen the crystal energy field by crisscrossing the light lines. Do this back and forth. For example:

Visualize an energy line coming out of the FRONT LEFT corner crystal (#1) and connecting with the REAR RIGHT corner crystal (#3). Then send the energy ray back to the LEFT FRONT crystal (#1) again. Now repeat the pattern for the remaining two crystals. The FRONT RIGHT corner crystal (#2) will connect with the LEFT REAR corner crystal (#4). Then return the light ray back to the RIGHT FRONT crystal (#2). (See diagram.)

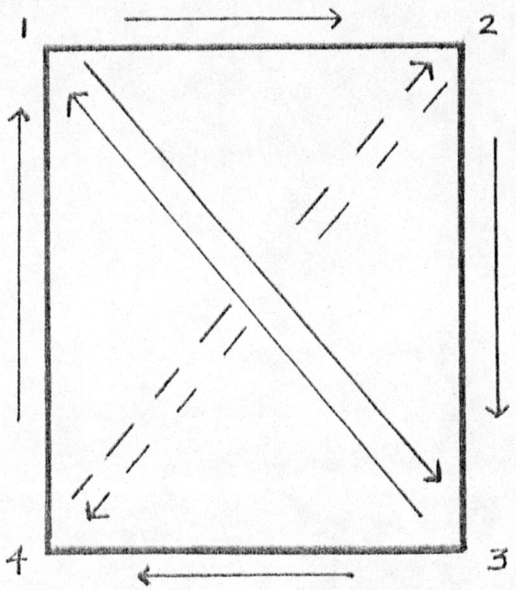

By connecting the crystals and light energy in this manner, you have created an etheric force field in which you are now going to bathe. Enjoy! Breathe in the Healing Light of the Universe. Upon completion dry off and if you feel guided, smudge yourself.

Now, recheck your energy readings with the Quartz Pendulum. If the energy centers register in a clockwise motion, then you are balanced out. They should be balanced. This is a powerful bath! It is good to check your chakras before and after this exercise. It shows you the difference in your energy patterns. If you can't work a pendulum, or you have a tendency to over influence it, then get a friend to measure you. They can use a pendulum or do muscle testing for each chakra center. I always feel like a new person after I take any of these crystal baths.

A final note : I do a clockwise motion over anything that I want to bless: food, bath water, charging crystal water, etc. I do a counter clockwise motion over anything when I want to clear the field. Some healers do this technique. Do what you feel guided to do.

MY PERSONAL EXPERIENCE:

EMOTIONAL RELEASING WITH CRYSTALS

After spending some time being exposed to different psychotherapeutic techniques, in particular, Re-evaluation Counseling, I have learned that it's okay to acknowledge our negative emotions. That it's important for us to allow them to surface so that we can release them and let them go. This can be a very transformative experience and it also creates a space inside our minds, so we can replace that area with some new input. I am a firm believer in releasing emotional issues. That is another book in the works. I also teach workshops on emotional healing.

At this time I'd like to share this exercise for emotional release. I call it the " Emotional Releaser ". It helps you to discharge unwanted thoughts and feelings. It helps you to release whatever emotions you need to look at and let go of.

The more I become involved in the healing arts, a healing channel, the more I am pressed to clean my own " house ". " Physician heal thyself." Daily we are all shown areas in our consciousness to work on and change. This is strongest in the area of relationships. I believe that there is a purpose to every person, place or thing. I don't believe in the term, " coincidence ". I believe in synchronicity. The synchronizing of the Universe.

Today, I am angry. Actually, I have been angry for a week now off and on with the anger peaking and subsiding. It depends on how much I allow this situation, this person to upset me. Here I am, a spiritual healer, and I'm not supposed to get upset with others. I am supposed to love everyone unconditionally. I know that, but I am also human.

So, now I need to look at why I am letting this person upset me. Because I believe in synchronicity and that everything has a purpose, I now need to recognize what this person is here to teach me. Everyone is our teacher. Everyone affects us. We are a summary of everyone we meet in life. We are all impressionable, but at different degrees.

So, why am I angry?

Why do I react to this person in this manner?

Why do I let this person upset me?

What part of her reflects a part of me that I don't like about myself?

Do I fear this person in any way? If so, why?

What are some nice qualities of this person?

How has this person benefited my life?

What have I learned from being exposed to this person?

When we recognize and allow negative emotions to surface and look at them, we can learn from them and grow. But, what do we do after we are done acknowledging them? We let go and go on with life. Here is a very powerful technique for releasing issues. It came to me while I was upset and needed to let go.

EMOTIONAL RELEASER

- Be seated in a quiet space. You may have a Meditation altar or table with a candle on it.

- Take a cleansed, large quartz crystal (about 1 - 1 1/2 lbs).

- Place the terminated end over the flame of a candle. Mentally clear and program your crystal. You can program it with the intention that the crystal will aid you in releasing emotional issues.

- Take the crystal into both hands and hold it at your chest level. Hold the termination end with the point directed upward.

- Do the Relaxation Breath. Inhale through your nostrils. Breathe in the Prana, the Life force of the Universe.

- Exhale out through your mouth.

- Direct your focus onto the crystal in your hands. This crystal is your tool for releasing. You are to put into it all negative, unwanted thought forms. All unwanted emotions. All unwanted memories. (It's okay. You will cleanse the crystal later when you are done.)

- Continue the Relaxation Breath.

- Exhale out of your mouth and breathe out into the crystal.

- Release into the crystal all ANGER. What color is your anger? Is it red? Project red (or another color that represents anger to you) into the crystal.

- Blow out hard. Exhale and get rid of that anger! Release ANGER from every cell in your body. Feel it leaving all parts of your body and going into the crystal. Pause for a minute.
If you feel like it, turn the crystal to another direction and blow onto another side, or facet of the crystal. After you fill up that facet, release into another facet and so on.

- Release FRUSTRATION. Let go of any frustration that you have been carrying around with you. Pause for a minute.

- Release any painful memories. Let them go now. Release the PAIN. Release the pain from every cell in your body. Pause for two minutes.

- Release any fears you have been holding onto. Let them go. Put them into the crystal.

- Let go of all negative emotions.

- Let go of all unwanted memories. Allow these to surface from every part of your being. Release these into the crystal. Fill the crystal. Pour out and release all unwanted memories into the crystal. Pause two minutes. You are ready to start anew and these negative thoughts and feelings have been holding you back. Let them all go NOW! Put them into the crystal NOW! Allow yourself to become free. You are worthy to be free and feel good about yourself. Don't let anything hold you back. LET IT ALL GO NOW!

- Now take a slow deep breath and yell out into the crystal. At the end of your " Yelling Chant " exhale hard from your diaphram. Repeat this three times. Do this until you feel you have completed your release discharge into the crystal. (Pause.) Now with all of your focus and might, breathe out hard one last time. This is your final victory of releasing the monster within. (Pause.)

- Take the crystal and place it over the candle with the terminated end pointed down towards the flame. Mentally clear your crystal.

- Now, go outside and bury the crystal. Bury what you have released into the ground. It will not harm Mother Earth. She can take the crystal and cleanse it. As you bury the crystal, remember that you are burying a part of your past self. You are symbolizing completely letting go of what you don't want and no longer need for your growth process.

You may want to keep the crystal buried in the earth for a full moon cycle. If you don't want it in the ground for that length of time, then at least keep it buried for a week. After you dig up the crystal you can re-use it, or if you feel guided, you can soak it in a salt water solution for a few days. It then is ready for any future time when you may need to release some other issues.

It is best to keep this crystal for this particular purpose: Emotional Releasing. As we go through life, we do accumulate mental / emotional "stuff" and this is a great way to release it. How do you feel? I feel great when I have done this technique!

Note: if you live in a city apartment, you can bury the crystal in a pot filled with dirt and use it only for this particular purpose. Occasionally, you can change the soil and throw out the old dirt. (As with any substance from the earth: sage, cedar, and dirt should be given back to Mother Earth. When you are done with your sacred herbs for smudging you should take them out to a field and either bury them or toss them on the ground. Don't throw them in the garbage. Respect that they have served you well. Dispose of them in a respectful manner.)

When people plant crystals in the ground, many plant them with the point up. Do as you feel guided to do.

MY PERSONAL EXPERIENCE:

BASIC ENERGY LAYOUTS WITH CRYSTALS

FOUR DIRECTIONS ENERGY LAYOUT

Supplies needed: Four palm size Clear Quartz Crystals.

This layout is used for meditations or charging objects.

Locate the true directions of the East, South, West and North. (Use a compass if you are unsure.)

Place each crystal in East, South, West and North directions. The terminated ends should be pointed in toward the center.

Sit in the center of the four crystals. Relax and center yourself. Sit in this crystal pattern for about fifteen to twenty minutes. If you feel guided, you can hold a quartz cluster in your hands. Sit in the direction you feel guided to face. Many sit facing the East. If you choose to lie down in this energy pattern, it is advised to have your head facing North. Your feet would be to the South. This flows with the polarities of the earth.

You can charge crystals, water, or other objects in this energy pattern. If you place charging objects inside a pyramid, this process would be amplified. The Four Direction layout could be either inside or outside the pyramid.

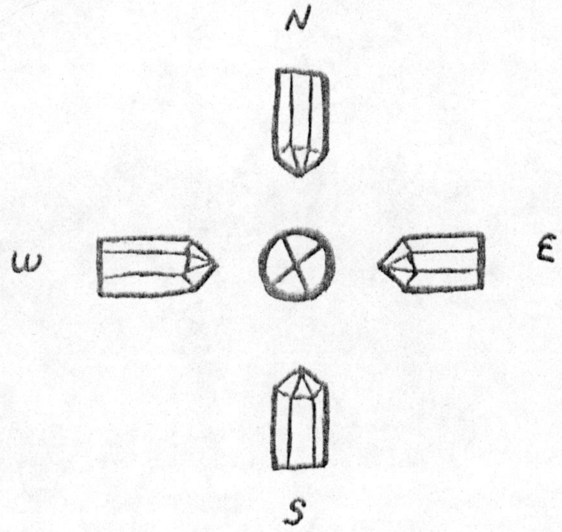

Other suggested crystal energy patterns are: Triangles, Six and Twelve Pointed Stars. See Exploring Atlantis, Vol. I by Dr. Frank Alper for these layouts.

MY PERSONAL EXPERIENCE:

CIRCLE PATTERN : for Multiple Balancings

This exercise aids in balancing all of the levels of our being, in particular the emotional level.

Supplies needed:

Thirteen Clear Quartz Crystals.

Thirteen Rose Quartz chunks or pebbles.

13 x 2 = 26   26 = 2 + 6 = 8   Eight is the number of balance, power and facilitation.

Place the crystals in a cirlce. Alternate one Clear Quartz and then one Rose Quartz until you have completed the cirlce. The Clear Quartz points should be aimed in toward the center of the circle.

This is a very powerful pattern. When you first do this crystal pattern, just sit in it for about fifteen to twenty minutes. After you have experienced the energy flow a few times, then experiment with bringing one or two crystals into your energy pattern with you.

MY PERSONAL EXPERIENCE:

CRYSTALS AND RADIESTHESIA

Pendulum dowsing was practiced in ancient civilizations. It was kept secret in the mystery schools until it reached Europe. It then became more common place and was used along with other dowsing techniques for locating: water, oil, minerals, and patient diagnosis. At the turn of this century, a French country priest by the name of Abbe Mermet coined the term, " radiesthesia ". He used dowsing for locating water, locating missing persons and for discovering diseases. (He even had the support of the Vatican behind him.) 2.

Here's how to do Pendulum dowsing:

Hold the pendulum in your dominant hand. (Use the hand that you write with.) Arch your wrist so that the cord is clasped between your thumb and forefinger. This way the pendulum will have a direct drop. Many people hold the string or cord about six to eight inches above the pendulum.

There are five basic movements to a pendulum:

1. Clockwise.

2. Counterclockwise.

3. Back and forth on the vertical.

4. Back and forth on the horizontal.

5. A diagonal leaning right or left.

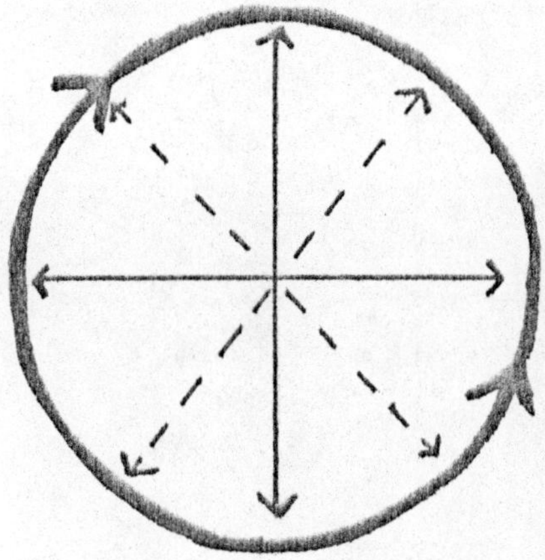

2. (The Science and Art of the Pendulum, Gabriele Blackburn, Idylwild Books, 1984).

Everyone's energy is different. For the majority of people, the " yes " answer is usually clockwise. The " no " answer can be counter-clockwise, back and forth or diagonal. You'll have to figure out for yourself which is your " yes " or " no " answer. You can do this by asking yes and no questions that you already know the answer to.

Dowsing Crystals

The Dowsing crystal that I am refering to is a natural Clear Quartz Crystal that is attached to a cord. I prefer a Quartz Pendulum over any other pendulum material because it has more benefits.

Since it is a quartz crystal, it amplifies the dowser's energy and consciousness.

It is beneficial in broadcasting light energy for Absentee Healings.

It is beneficial in emitting light energy for healing sessions with clients.

It can be programmed and used to channel a specific color or energy vibration for multiple purposes.

The list is endless. When I do any dowsing work with pendulums, I mostly use natural quartz crystals. Dowsing crystals can be used for: Absentee Healing, locating energy blockages and for energy balancing.

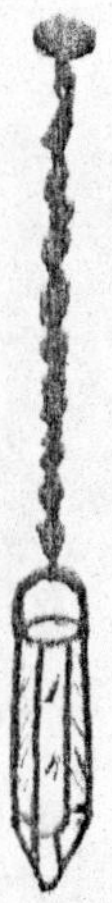

A Dowsing Crystal

ADDITIONAL USES

Clearing an Energy Field:

Swing a dowsing crystal in a counterclockwise motion until it stops. This can be done over food, crystal bath waters, photographs, or in session work. If a client has an imbalanced area, you can clear the area with a counterclockwise motion before doing any other balancing work.

Balancing an Energy Field - " Energy Blessing ":

Swing the dowsing crystal in a clockwise motion until it stops. To add to this process, you can put your empty hand up towards the Heavens and fill up your open palm with healing light energy. Channel this cosmic energy throughout your body and down through the pendulum into the rotating crystal.

If you do not have a dowsing crystal, then you can use a single point crystal or your hands. You will achieve the same results. Counter-clockwise motion represents energy that is transformative and con-centrated. It clears and balances an object. Clockwise motion represents energy that is expansive. These are not the same as in reading energy imbalances. Please refer to the section on, " How to Measure Energy ". This topic is also discussed in advanced classes and will be mentioned in a future book.

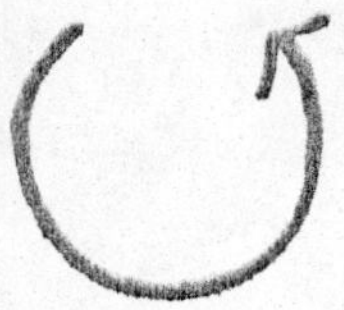

Concentrated

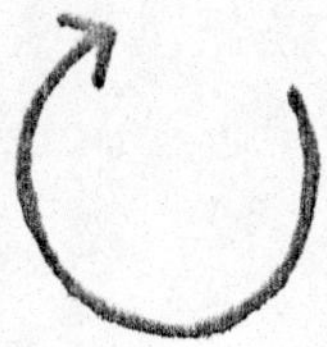

Expansive

THE CHAKRAS: OUR ENERGY CENTERS

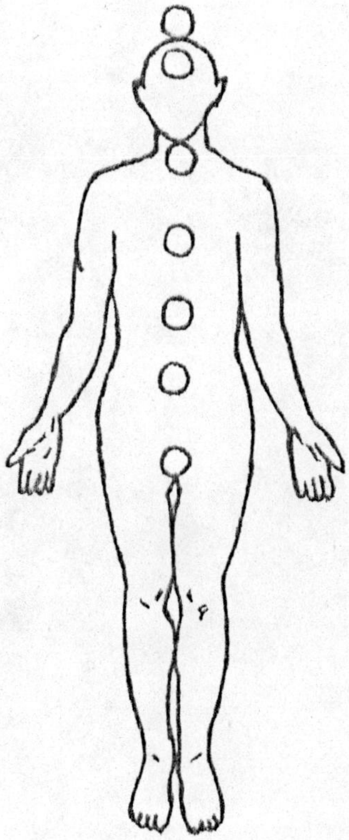

The word chakra means wheel. The chakras are revolving vortices of spiritual energy existing in the subtle bodies. They relate to major nerve plexuses, glands and organs in the physical body. The chakras are the interchange points of energy between the physical and the super-physical aspects of human nature. They link the subtle bodies and project energy into and receive energy from the outside environment. 1.

Chakras are located in the area of a nerve plexus. Most of the points of the Meridian System (Acupuncture / Acupressure) relate specifically to one of the Major or Minor chakras.

STONES FOR BALANCING THE CHAKRA CENTERS

Below:

Black & Brown stones: Obsidian, Smoky Quartz, Black Tourmaline, Black Onyx and Apache Tears (Obsidian). These are used for grounding energy and becoming " rooted " with the earth. This is important for a proper energy flow.

First Chakra:

Ruby, Garnet, Red Jasper, Bloodstone. These stones represent the the RED color ray, which is associated with the ROOT Chakra.

Second Chakra:

Carnelian, Madiera Citrine (Quartz). These represent the ORANGE color ray.

Third Chakra:

Golden Topaz, Golden Citrine, Amber, Golden Calcite. These represent the YELLOW color ray.

1. Survival Into the 21st Century, by Viktoras Kulvinskas, Omangod Press, P.O. Box 255, Wethersfield, Conn. 06109.

Fourth Chakra:

Green: Green Tourmaline, Emerald, Malachite, Peridot, Green Garnet, Chrysoprase, Dioptase, green Jade, Adventurine and Watermelon Tourmaline.

Pink: Rose Quartz, Kunzite, Rhodochrosite, Rubellite (pink Tourmaline),pink Jade and Watermelon Tourmaline. Both the colors GREEN and PINK balance the HEART Center. (This is the center of love and compassion. Pink is the color of unconditional love.)

Fifth Chakra:

Aquamarine, Turquoise, Chrysocolla, blue Tourmaline, blue Lace Agate, Celestite, Amazonite and blue Topaz. These represent the BLUE color ray.

Sixth Chakra:

Sodalite, Lapis Lazuli, Sapphire, and Azurite. These represent dark blue - INDIGO color ray.

Seventh Chakra:

Amethyst, Alexandrite, purple Fluorite and Sugilite (Royal Azel). These represent the VIOLET color ray.

Above the head - Transpersonal Point:

Calcite, Clear Quartz and Diamond. This represents the WHITE ray. White contains all of the color spectrum.

THE CHAKRA ENERGY SYSTEM

# / NAME	ANTERIOR LOCATION	BALANCING COLOR	BALANCING NOTE	ELEMENT	ENDOCRINE ASSOCIATION	NERVE PLEXUS	POSTERIOR LOCATION	ESOTERIC RELATIONSHIP TO THE CENTERS
Major Chakras:								
1. Root / Base Center	Base of the Spine	RED	C	EARTH	Gonads	Coccygeal	4th Sacral Vertebra	Physical Activity Stability, Survival
2. Spleen / Navel Center	Lower Abdomen Below Navel	ORANGE	D	WATER	Pancreas	Splenic	1st Lumber Vertebra	Feelings, Sensations Creativity
3. Solar Plexus	Between Navel & base of Sternum	YELLOW	E	FIRE	Adrenals	Solar / Coeliac Plexus	8th Thoracic Vertebra	Personal Power Will
4. Heart Center	Center of Chest	GREEN	F	AIR	Thymus	Cardiac	1st Thoracic Vertebra	Love, Compassion Healing
5. Throat Center	Middle of Throat	BLUE	G	ETHER	Thyroid / Parathyroid	Pharyngeal	3rd Cervical Vertebra	Communication Self Expression
6. Brow Center	Between Eyebrows	INDIGO	A	-	Pituitary	Carotid	1st Cervical Vertebra	Visualization (Clairvoyance) Perception
7. Crown Center	Top of Head	VIOLET	B	-	Pineal	Brain Dendrites	None	Liberation Cosmic Consciousness
Transpersonal Point	12-24" above Head	WHITE	ALL SOUND	-	-	-	-	Divine Connection

Minor Chakras:

Feet, Ankles, Calves, Knees, Hips, Pelvic Girdle, Hands, Wrists, Forearms, Elbows and Shoulders.

How to Measure Energy Centers

You can locate energy blockages by passing a pendulum over the surface of the body. This applies in particular with the Major and Minor Chakra locations. If the pendulum swings counterclockwise then there is an imbalance. You can also touch an area with one hand while you hold the pendulum in the other hand. The results should be the same. Another way to locate energy blockages is to do Applied Kinesiology, muscle testing. This technique involves two people. One person is the " tester". The client extends an arm straight out at shoulder level. The tester applies gentle pressure at the client's forearm. The motion is downward, while the client tries to resist that motion. The arm should feel like it has " locked " in place and has resisted the tester's pressure. This would be refered to as, a " positive response". If the client's arm does not " lock " into place, then the arm will follow through in a downward motion. This is refered to as, a " negative response". Muscle testing is a fine art and takes a lot of practice.

By muscle testing or dowsing, you can locate a client's energy blockages, find out which vitamins and minerals are missing in his / her diet, and also what substances the client is allergic to. Many chiropractors use Applied Kinesiology in their session work.

Whether you use a pendulum or do muscle testing, you should get the same results and answers. These techniques when done properly are addressing the Higher Self (superconscious) of a person. It is from that place that we are guided to do what is good for us.

Measuring the Chakras

See the Chakra Location Chart.

Pendulum Method:

Client can be standing, sitting, or lying down.

Center yourself. Do the Relaxation Breath. You need to be relaxed, centered and clear so that you don't influence the pendulum reading.

Place the pendulum in the location of a chakra area. Mentally ask yourself, " What is the energy of this person's (name) chakra center?" Observe which direction the pendulum swings. Clockwise (balanced) or counterclockwise (not balanced).

Many practitioners do Chakra readings from the Base chakra to the Crown Chakra. Start at the Base and then measure the Spleen, then the Solar Plexus, Heart, Throat, Brow and lastly, the Crown Chakra. (This is different in a general energy reading, such as Therapeutic Touch. In that case, practitioners use their hands and scan from the head down to the feet.)

Go through and measure all of the Major Chakra centers. Next measure the elbows, hands, knees and feet.

If you have learned the Therapeutic Touch technique then you can do a body scan (patient assesstment); then recheck with the pendulum.

You can also recheck your readings by muscle testing in relation to the chakra areas.

For measuring your own centers, you can use a pendulum. When you get to the top centers, measure them in front of a mirror. (It helps you from going cross-eyed.)

Applied Kinesiology Method:

It helps to have both the client and the tester relaxed and centered. This way there is less of a possibility of influencing the reading.

For muscle testing, the client is usually standing. You also can test someone who is lying down. If they are bed ridden and weak, you'll need to do surrogate testing.

Place your LEFT hand over the client's chakra area and muscle test the arm. Does it lock or does it feel weak and follow through on your downward motion? If the arm locks, the chakra is balanced. Go through and measure the other centers in the same manner. (Remember a lot of people do not test true with muscle testing. They over compensate their muscles and then end up testing strong on everything. It's like you get a " Muscle Beach " response. This goes for women, as well as men. What about people who study martial arts? Forget it! They really know how to center and focus their energy.)

When you do locate energy imbalances with either of these methods, then the next step is to choose a Crystal Healing Meditation exercise. Upon completion recheck the energy centers. They should balance out.

If Applied Kinesiology interests you and you would like to go further with it, I highly recommend taking some courses. For more information, you can contact:

TOUCH FOR HEALTH FOUNDATION
1174 North Lake Ave.
Pasadena, Calif. 91104

(213) 794-1181

They offer international training seminars in Touch For Health and Edu-Kinesthetics. They also have a referral service of instructors who may be located in your area.

There are several ways to balance the Chakra Centers. This is also the case in the therapeutic application of crystals. Here is one suggested way:

CRYSTAL CHAKRA MEDITATION FOR BALANCING

Supplies needed:

Eight or nine palm size Clear Quartz Crystals (These should weigh about 8 ounces each.)

Two Generator Clear Quartz Crystals. (These should be larger than the other crystals.)

Find a quiet space. Place all of the crystals within arm's reach and lie down. (If possible, have your head pointing North and your feet South.)

Place one Generator Crystal above your head. Point the terminated end towards your head.

Place one Generator Crystal below your feet. Point the terminated end towards your feet and legs.

Take the remaining crystals and place one on each of the Chakra Centers. Begin at the Base, Spleen / Navel, Solar Plexus, Heart, Throat, Brow and Crown. (Place the heavier ones on the chakras located below the throat.)

Place the remaining two crystals in your hands. The LEFT hand will hold the crystal with the point aimed at the shoulders. The RIGHT hand will hold the crystal with the point aimed away from the body.

Note: The crystal for the Crown Chakra can be turned sideways and placed along the top of the head. You could also leave it out and use the Generator Crystal to represent the Crown Chakra Crystal. If you are working with seven programmed chakra crystals that have been attuned with the appropriate colors and sounds, then you will be using all seven. (See the section on programming crystals.) Some practitioners place the Crown Chakra Crystal with the point up, while others, point it down. Do what you feel guided to do.

You are now ready to begin. Close your eyes and quiet your mind. Do the Relaxation Breath. Allow yourself to relax and deepen. Ground yourself by visualizing that you are growing luminous roots into the earth. Allow your energies to mingle with the energies of Mother Earth. Pause for two minutes.

Visualize the color vibration of RED coming up out of the earth. See the color traveling to the base of your spine. As the red ball of energy begins to balance your Base Chakra Center, it becomes more vivid in color. Sense it balancing and strengthening this area. Pause for three minutes.

Visualize the color ORANGE coming up out of the earth. See the color traveling to your lower abdomen area. See the orange balancing and strengthening this area. Pause for two minutes.

Visualize the color YELLOW coming up out of the earth. See the color traveling to your solar plexus area. See yellow balancing and strengthening this area. Pause for two minutes.

Visualize the color GREEN in the distance. See it horizontal and parallel above the ground. Draw in this healing energy to the center of your chest. See green balancing your Heart Chakra Area. This is the meeting place of the Lower and Upper Chakras. See this area being strengthened. Pause for two to three minutes.

Bring the remaining colors in from the Heavens:

Visualize the color BLUE traveling down from the Heavens. See the color entering and filling up your throat area. This is the Center of Communication and Expression. See blue balancing and strengthening this area. Pause for two minutes.

Visualize the color INDIGO traveling down from the Heavens. See the color entering and filling up your brow area. See indigo balancing and strengthening your Brow Chakra. Pause for two minutes.

Visualize the color VIOLET traveling down from the Heavens. See the color entering and filling up the top of your head. Violet is the color of transmutation. See violet balancing and strengthening your Crown Chakra. Pause for two minutes.

Visualize a ball of light about eighteen inches above your head area. This area represents your Transpersonal Point. It connects you with the Universe. See golden light balancing and amplifying this area. Sense your Divine Connection. Pause for three minutes.

Take the Crown Chakra Crystal and place it in your RIGHT hand. Point the terminated end away from the body. Use your crystal and draw a line connecting your chakras together. Begin with the Transpersonal Point and connect it with your Crown Chakra. Touch the point of the crystal to the chakra centers as you connect them together. Next, connect the Crown Chakra to the Brow Chakra. Again, touch the crystal points directly to the chakra areas. Next, connect the Brow Chakra to the Throat Chakra. Continue this until you have drawn a crystal connection from the Crown to the Base Chakra.

When you have completed doing this, place the crystal at your head space. Continue to rest in the crystal energy field with all of the chakra crystals in place. Be sensitive to your own energy. Most people who do this exercise average about ten to thirty minutes in being exposed to the crystals in this manner.

Remove the crystals and rest for another ten minutes. This helps you to adjust to any energy changes you may experience. This crystal exercise charges you. You may feel more energetic. It amplifies your energy field. One way to prove this is to have another person dowse your energy field. This can be done with a Cameron Aurameter, or Angle Rods. They can reveal the distance of of how far your energy field emanates. (These items in particular can be ordered from the American Dowsing Society. See the back of this book for the address.)

If you feel somewhat lightheaded after doing this exercise, then hold your feet and ground your energies. Visualize growing luminous roots into the earth. This will direct your energies down. Sometimes we get headaches or feel lightheaded because there is too much energy in our head space.

After you have done this crystal exercise a few times, introduce some music into this meditation. Steven Halpern's " Spectrum Suite " (the short version) can be used for balancing the chakras. Whether you use crystals or not, you can balance the chakras with color visualizations and the music of this tape. If you are working with chakra crystals that have been programmed with the music of this tape, it will be more effective during your balancings.

MY PERSONAL EXPERIENCE:

SESSION WORK

SESSION SHEETS

Before I do session work on my clients, I first do an Energy Assessment. Also, if it is the first time that I will work with someone, then I will take a short client history at the initial visit. This can be very helpful. One time I was with a client who had not given me a complete medical report. At one point he began to act peculiar. Within a matter of seconds he was on the floor going into a Grand Mal Seizure and convulsing. I have had ambulance and emergency room experience in the past, so I was able to handle the situation well. Someone else may have panicked in this situation. As it turned out, the client was an epileptic and had not taken his medication for a couple of days. (It pays to know first aid. Contact your local American Red Cross for basic instruction in first aid and CPR.)

Another reason to take some notice of your client's medical condition, would be in the case of pacemakers. I do not use Crystal Therapy on <u>any</u> client who is wearing a pacemaker. Crystals emit an energy vibration. That particular vibration may alter the rhythm of the pacemaker. Heart conditions are a touchy situation. Laying on of hands is sufficient. Know CPR (Cardio Pulmonary Resuscitation). What would you do if your client had a heart attack while you were in session together? How would you handle it?

Another reason to keep session reports is that it will show the progress or decline pattern of a client. You will also have a comparison of notes from one session to another. This can be a valuable aid for you. If you use a few different healing modalities, then you can keep better track of what you've used in the past. You can also keep track of which crystal techniques you have used, along with which particular crystals and gemstones were applied in session work.

The more time you spend in the beginning keeping notes on your session work, the better you will become. It is like journal writing. Each time you review the sessions, you'll see it with different eyes and perception. Here are some session sheets that I use in session work.:

Sheet # 1 - Initial Client Information Sheet:

This gives you a brief medical history of the client. It also informs you about any medications the client may be presently taking. (You can purchase a PDR - Physician's Desk Reference if you want to look up medication information. It gives you an idea of what the client is on and why his or her doctor prescribed it.)

The body and mind store much information. In particular they can recall trauma that has taken place in the past. This can be from operations or accidents, for example. In doing spiritual healing work with the application of crystals many avenues can be explored. The patient may get in touch with unresolved issues that relate on a physical, emotional, mental or spiritual level. If the healing practitioner is aware about certain issues ahead of time; he or she may be able to assist the client better as the releasing arises. (This is not absolutely necessary, but it helps.)

Sheet # 2 - Session Intake Sheet:

This sheet lists the physical, emotional, mental and spiritual levels of the client. It helps the client to focus attention upon these areas. The client expresses the present state of condition for each level and also what he or she would like to change. This opens up communication between the client and the holistic practitioner. Many issues that normally would not be expressed may get a chance to be discussed.

It is suggested that the Session Intake Sheet be filled out on each visit. We are all constantly evolving. Each day we are given new experiences to assist us in our growth process. If you have returning clients, your intake sheets will help to record any significant changes.

Initial Client Information Sheet

Date ___/___/___

Name ______________________________ Phone ____________________

Address _______________________City / State __________________ Zip___

Significant Medical History:

Are you presently under the supervision of a doctor?

Doctor's name and address:

Are you presently taking any medications? If so, please list.

Please list any operations you have had in the past.

Please list any major accidents you have had in the past.

What is your reason for coming here today?

Session Intake Sheet

Date ___/___/___

Name ______________________________ Phone ___________________________

Describe your present conditions of the following areas. Also, explain what you would like to change about them.

PHYSICAL:

EMOTIONAL:

MENTAL:

SPIRITUAL:

Why are you here today?

Sheet # 3: Session Sheets

These sheets are used for each session to record the following:

Energy assessments of the client.

Specific healing modalities used during the session.

Specific crystals and gemstones used and their exact locations during the session.

Time session lasted.

Reassessment of client's energy.

1: Therapeutic Touch Assessment. This is directed to those who are trained in this technique. The practitioner uses his or her hands to scan the energy field of the client. They assess the energy levels from head to feet.

2: Chakra Assessment. Read the article on " How to Measure the Energy Centers ". You will circle the imbalanced centers on the session sheet.

3: This is for listing various techniques used during the session. For example: one time I used Therapeutic Touch, Reiki Healing, Crystal Healing and Guided Imagery during session work. Another time, I might use Reiki Healing and Essence Counseling. It's important to keep a record of what was done during the session.

4 & 5: During table work, the client may be surrounded with crystals. You may also place some on different areas of the body. Different locations and different minerals will yield different results. It is important to keep a good description of your different crystal placements and methods used. You will learn from them as you do them and also review them. We learn from our experiences.

6: Some sessions may be more significant than others.

7: It helps to stay in touch with the needs of each client. Each person is an unique individual with a specific need that arises at any given moment.

8: Reassess the client's energy field. This way you will have a comparison with before and after the session work.

9: It's good to keep track of your session time. You may start out in the beginning of your practice with disorientation of time. I average one and a half to two hours with each client. The first half hour includes assessment, Therapeutic Touch and some relaxation techniques. The following hour or hour and a half involves the table work. It helps to be aware of time so you don't spend too much time in one area and neglect another area of the body. One half hour on the front and one half hour on the back is a good average. Some may spend less time with their clients. Many holistic practitioners charge by the hour for their work. That is a standard procedure. If you plan to work on a few clients on the same day, you don't want to overlap one session with another. There should be a ten minute resting period after the balancing session. This allows the client time to adjust to any energy changes that may have occurred during the session.

10: Keep track of what tapes you played during the session. It's nice to offer a variety for returning clients.

Session Sheet

Name________________________________ Date ___/___/___.

Phone____________________________ Starting Time ____:____

1: Therapeutic Touch Assessment: ______________________________

____

____

____

2: Chakra Assessment: ____

____

____

<u>Circle</u> chakra imbalances: Base Navel / Spleen

Solar Plexus Heart Throat Brow Crown

elbows palms knees feet

3: List techniques used during the session.

Additional notes:

4: Session layout for crystal work: Mark your placement locations and list crystals and gemstones used during the session.

FRONT BACK

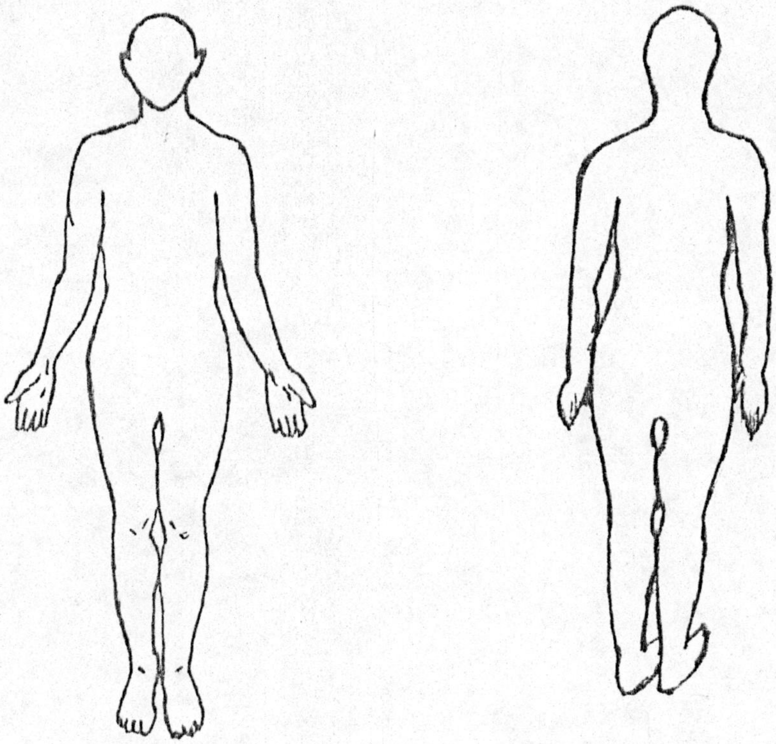

Additional notes:

5: Table work:

Techniques applied: ____

____

____

6: List significant occurrences during the session.

7: Describe what your client's needs were during the session.

After Session:

8: Energy Reassessment: ____________________________________

____

____

9: Time of session work: ___________________________________

Table work time: ____

Total time: ____

10: Relaxation tapes played: ______________________________

____

____

Notes on Session Work:

Use only Clear Quartz Crystal through the energy field.

You can use any Fluorite in an area along side of another crystal or gemstone. The Fluorite should be removed after twelve to fifteen minutes. Its purpose is to open up the pathway for crystals and gemstones. It clears the energy field of an area.

You can use specific stones in certain areas for balancing. See the listings on " Spiritual Medicine Chest " and " Stones for Balancing the Chakras ".

Everyone's energy is different. Some clients will be more sensitive than others. Stay in tune with your client's needs.

There are many possible crystal patterns and layouts for Crystal Healing. The chart on the following page is an example of a session layout.

General Layout of Crystals & Gemstones during Session Work

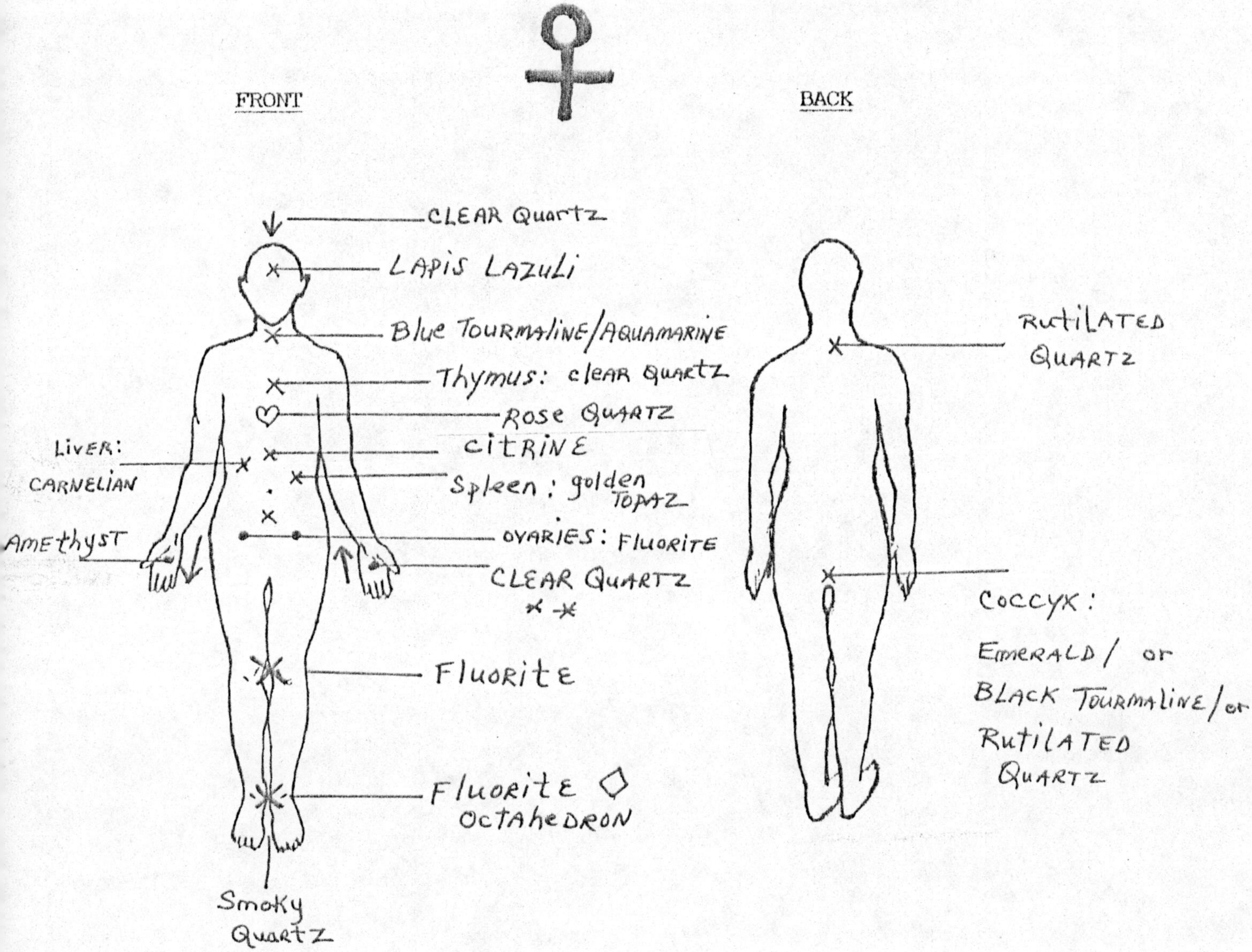

* Ⓛ HAND ALTERNATIVES: AQUAMARINE (STRESS); Rhodochrosite (emotional issues); LEPIDOLITE (DEPRESSION); etc.

HEALING THERAPIES AND THE USE OF CRYSTALS

REIKI & CRYSTALS

Reiki (ray-key) is an ancient healing art rediscovered in Japan in the late 1800's by Dr. Mikao Usui. Reiki is a Japanese word meaning Universal Life Energy, the energy that is all around us. Reiki goes beyond being just another healing art. It also involves spiritual initiations that are given by a Reiki Master to the student. Each Reiki initiation involves a level of energy transference between the Reiki Master and the initiate. These transferences of energy that the students are attuned to reawakens and reopens their healing channel.

There are four levels in Reiki Healing.

First Degree: Practitioner has learned specific hand positions for doing energy work that helps to balance a person's physical, etheric, emotional, mental and spiritual levels.

Second Degree: Practitioner is able to do the same as a First Degree with the addition of: The ability to do advanced methods of mental / emotional healings and the ability to do healings at a distance (absentee healings). They are also trained in using powerful energy symbols that activate these processes.

Third Degree: Reiki Master. Can do the same as First and Second Degrees with the addition of: The ability to initiate and activate another's healing channel for First and Second Degree levels.

Fourth Degree: Reiki Grandmaster. One who has the ability to initate a Reiki Master. The current Grandmaster of Reiki is Phyllis Lei Furumoto, who resides in Santa Fe, New Mexico.

In this section, I will address the First and Second Degree levels of Reiki Healing and the use of quartz crystals. I find that adding crystals to my Reiki Healing sessions accentuates the energy work.

Here are a few things that seem to consistently occur when crystals are added to Reiki Healing:

The time spent doing hand positions in a particular area is shortened.

The client's awareness and sensitivity to the balancings is increased.

The client's responses are more accentuated: releasing, discharging, opening of congested areas are often times dramatic.

The client's recovery time for healing is accelerated.

Here are some suggestions for using crystals in your Reiki practice and also on yourself:

Reiki on Yourself:

Much of my free time in bed, I do Reiki Healing on myself. Before I get out of bed in the morning and before I go to sleep, I practice Reiki. It helps me to drift off to sleep more than other nights. It is hard to do Reiki on your own back. To reach around and get your open palm over certain places is not an easy task. I have found Herkimer Diamonds excellent in helping out in this situation. For example, my schedule gets hectic at times. It causes me to race around, which in turn drains my energy, especially in the adrenal and kidney areas. I can feel it and at times the energy is so blocked that there is pain there. Here's what I do for it:

I place a Herkimer (palm size or smaller) underneath my back over one kidney area. It is left there for about five to ten minutes. I move it to the adrenal area next. Whatever aches the most gets first priority. Then after one side feels completed, I move the crystal over to the other side which is underneath my back at the kidney, and later at the adrenal area. While the crystal is underneath my back, I am resting face up. I visualize healing light energy being released from the Herkimer crystal into that imbalanced area of my body. I also can be doing Reiki on my front positions while the crystal is balancing out my back. I have found this to work every time.

Reiki on Yourself:

You can hold one crystal in each hand and do Reiki on your front and head positions. Note: Holding crystals while doing Reiki is different from described elsewhere. Since you are attuned to a specific vibration of the Universal Flow, the energy is directed out of both hands. In this case, the crystals in both hands should be pointed outward towards your finger tips and away from the body.

You can rest your back on two crystals and while they balance out different back positions, you can be doing Reiki on your front postions.

Reiki on Others:

First Degree:

You can hold a crystal in each hand while doing Reiki on another person. Again, the crystals should be pointed towards your finger tips and away from the body.

You can place crystals or gemstones on particular body positions and then place your hands (without crystals) over those areas.

You can place crystals and gemstones on a client's body in a particular location, while you are doing Reiki elsewhere on his or her body, especially Fluorite or quartz crystals. These will open up the congested areas. When you get to those areas to do Reiki, you'll have a head start. The Reiki Healing will go further inside the body and be more effective.

Reiki on Yourself & Others:

Second Degree:

Mental / Emotional Healings: Place crystals in your hands and do the Mental Healing positions. The CROWN crystal should be pointed towards the front of the body. The crystal in the other hand should be pointed up.

Absentee Healings: You can place Reiki programmed crystals onto photographs of the people you are sending healing energy to.

You can program all of your jewelry with the powerful Reiki symbols. This will charge your crystal jewelry. You can also do this for your other crystals. Remember that if you cleanse your crystals in saltwater you will erase their programs. Just program them again with the Reiki symbols.

Reiki on Others:

Second Degree:

You can draw Reiki energy symbols with palm size Clear Quartz Crystals. This can be done over a photograph, your food, or a client's body, to name a few .

You can draw the energy symbols with your hands and direct that energy into a quartz crystal. You would be programming Reiki Energy symbols into it for later use.

You can program crystals with the Reiki symbols and give them to your friends and clients. These will serve as attunement instruments for your later use of doing distant healings on them. The crystals need to be in their aura (energy field), such as in a pocket, or worn around their neck, or tied to their bed, if they are bedridden.

First and Second Degrees:

You can also program a crystal with the Reiki Initiation energy. Some Reiki Masters do not permit the wearing of a quartz crystal during the energy transferences, because the Reiki energy is too powerful. So, if you are not permitted to wear it, you could still have it in the room during the spiritual initiations. This way, when you meditate, you can recall that experience. It will be stored in the crystal. If you feel close to your Reiki Master, you can have a crystal with your teacher's energy in it. Just have him or her say a blessing into it.

For more information on Reiki Healing, or if you would like to locate a Reiki Master in your area, write to:

The Reiki Alliance
535 Cordova Road, Suite # 419
Santa Fe, New Mexico 87501

(505) 983-8659

This is an international organization that offers Reiki training in most parts of the world.

If you are located in the Northeast of the U.S., contact:

Ojela Frank
c/o The Holistic Health Works
P.O. Box 327-CTB
New City, N.Y. 10956

I keep track of which Reiki Masters of the Reiki Alliance are available in various locations.

May blessings of Reiki be with you.

MariEl Healing and Crystals

MariEl Healing is a New Age healing art. It also invloves spiritual attunements and energy transferences. As of this writing, there are only two MariEl Masters who can channel the MariEl Energy for initiations. They are the founder, Ethel Lombardi and her assistant, Shirley Hortzman.

I met Ethel Lombardi in the summer of 1983 at a Life Spectrum Seminar. We only met for a few moments. It was enough time to know that she is a very special woman. I have studied with many healers and spiritual teachers. No one has touched me that intensely in an initial meeting. When you look into the eyes of Ethel Lombardi, you see only one thing, unconditional love. Here I was with this stranger, this powerful woman and I was completely overwhelmed. I looked back into her eyes and said, " We will meet again. " We had bonded together as one in just a brief moment of our existence together. Amazing!

I had the opportunity to study with Ethel for her MariEl training and then in an advanced class. From my exposure to Ethel, I have come to the conclusion that Ethel Lombardi truly channels the energy of the Divine Mother. She does not advertise what she channels. You have to figure that out for yourself.

The key to MariEl Healing is that it involves heart to heart and Higher Self to Higher Self. It focuses on emotional healing and emotional releasing. If you ever take a class of any sort with Ethel, I highly recommend that you bring a box of Kleenex with you. You'll thank me for it. You end up releasing a lot of emotional issues around that lady.

Within my first few months of doing MariEl Healing in my holistic practice, I found it was a key for doing Past Life Regression (PLR) therapy. By using crystals, anointing oils, some PLR visualizations along with the MariEl energy in session work, the results would sometimes get amazingly interesting. Not only would the clients be going into past lives, but I would also be able to assist them in healing those past lives. This would be achieved with the MariEl releasing techniques.

MariEl Healing is not only for PLR therapy. You cannot guarantee that every client will be able to achieve PLR with you. Only the ones who are really ready will be able to experience it.

I only did PLR therapy in the beginning of my MariEl session work. In recent years, I have gone back to doing mostly Reiki Healing in my sessions. But, I feel that those who are actively using MariEl in their session work deserve some recognition for Ethel's sharing. Here are some suggestions for using crystals in MariEl Healing:

Drawing the energy lines can be more effective if you are holding quartz crystals. Or you can draw the lines <u>with</u> them. Note: when holding crystals in your hands as a MariEl channel, the crystals should be pointed toward your finger tips away from the body.

Another suggestion is to place several crystals at the intersecting points of each energy line. You could also place crystals on each of the chakras (with the points aimed at the top of the head). This could be done while you are drawing the energy lines on a client who is lying down.

Because MariEl energy works so strongly with emotional issues and releasing, I am drawn to using many of the pink crystals and gemstones: Rose Quartz, Rhodochrosite, Rubellite (pink tourmaline) and Kunzite. MariEl energy is about unconditional love. That Love vibration is pink.

In the releasing technique and cutting etheric cords, you could use a crystal in each hand. The receiving hand (usually the left) could collect what the client is releasing, while the other hand is stirring up what needs to be released. This takes place over the heart, throat, or navel areas the most. Be sure to not use the collecting crystal at any other time in the session once the client has released into it. You don't want to put that "stuff" back into his or her energy field. Cleanse it in saltwater for a full week.

Some quartz and gemstone eggs are good for collecting into. Rose Quartz, Rhodochrosite and Clear Quartz are a few that I use. Or you could have the client hold them during the session, especially the pink ones.

For more information about taking classes with Ethel Lombardi or Shirley Hortzman, write to:

MariEl Seminars
Ethel Lombardi
93 Spring Creek Rd. Rte. 5
Lockport, Ill. 60441

(815) 838-8218

Ethel also teaches MariEl at the Edgar Cayce center during the summer months. Write to:

Assoc. for Research and Enlightenment
P.O. Box 595
Virginia Beach, Va. 23451

For more information on classes in the Northeast U.S. contact:

Ojela Frank
c/o The Holistic Health Works
P.O. Box 327-CTB
New City, N.Y. 10956

Therapeutic Touch and Crystals

God bless Dolores Krieger. If it hadn't been for her, everytime I go into a hospital to do spiritual healings, I'd get harassed. Now, all I have to say is Therapeutic Touch. Most of the nursing staff have heard of this at one point of their training or work space. Most nurses do welcome any extra attention that is given to their patients. They usually have a heavy work load schedule which limits their free time for additional patient care.

Therapeutic Touch is a technique that is derived from the laying on of hands, as described in the Bible. It goes beyond the laying on of hands. One who takes training in this technique learns about the concept of a universal life force. They learn how to relax, center, focus and transfer healing energies. We have discussed most of this in my book, but these concepts are a big idea for the medical field. Dr. Krieger has personally trained over four thousand health professionals in a fifteen year period. We needed this to occur and she was one of the pioneers and keys for opening up this pathway. It is a big step when the "N.Y. Times" finally gets around to mentioning the idea of Therapeutic Touch, as they did in a Spring '86 issue.

For more information about the Therapeutic Touch technique, I recommend Dr. Krieger's book, The Therapeutic Touch. (We carry it.) Also you can write to the suggested addresses at the end of this book. If you live in the N.Y.C. area, you're in luck! Janet Macrae, Ph.D and Dolores Krieger, Ph.D both teach Therapeutic Touch at New York University.

For now, I have a few suggestions for using crystals in a Therapeutic Touch session.

Patient Assessment: Scanning the energy field. Most T.T. practitioners first scan the energy field of a client before doing any balancing work.

You could hold a crystal in each hand while doing a patient assessment. The crystals will help to accentuate where the imbalances are located. (The crystal in the left hand has the point aimed towards the shoulders. The crystal in the right hand has the point aimed at the finger tips.)

For clients who are seated: During balancing work, you can place a large Fluorite Octahedron and / or a Smoky Quartz at the feet. This will assist in opening up the foot chakras and grounding the client's energy. It also helps to have the feet touching the crystal.

The client could be holding a crystal in each hand. The LEFT hand would hold a Clear Quartz with the point aimed at the client's shoulders. The RIGHT hand could hold an Amethyst or Clear Quartz Crystal with the point aimed towards the finger tips.

Therapeutic Touch practitioners could have a crystal in each hand during balancing work. This amplifies the energy that they are transfering to the client, or from one body area to another body location. Example: Sending energy from the shoulder to the wrist.

Brushing down the energy field with a crystal in your hand(s). The side of the crystal would be parallel with the client's body.

For clients who are lying down: Place Smoky Quartz or a large Fluorite Octahedron at the feet.

Client can be holding crystals or gemstones in both hands.

While you are working on one area of the body, you could place crystals and Fluorites in other locations. These will help to open up congested areas. It's like having a second set of healing hands!

If you are a nurse in a hospital setting and are not able to use crystals for whatever reason, you can wear a crystal pendant. This will help you to amplify your thoughts. Energy follows thought. As you make physical contact with your patients, your efforts will be amplified.

You could also obtain a mineral pouch and place a crystal inside of it. The crystal could be programmed for a specific patient and for a specific purpose. You then could give it as a gift, or a good luck token for his or her operation and speedy recovery. It could be tied to the bed frame. As long as it's in the patient's energy field, it will help them.

Many patients who have had quartz crystals on them during surgery and immediately there after, have had accelerated recovery times.

Absentee Healing

There is no limit to time and space in healing work. It involves working with the Life Force of the Universe, which has no limits. Long Distance Healing (also known as, Absentee Healing) is practiced by many throughout the world. It can be done in the form of prayer, meditation, crystal applications, Radionics, Psychotronics, or specific healing methods, as in Reiki or MariEl Healing. All of these methods work for one specific reason. Energy follows thought. By thinking and projecting a healing thought into the Universe, you are setting this motion into action. Many of us have heard of " miracles " occurring in reference to others being healed. I also have experienced this from my own applications. There is no mystery around distant healing. If a person is meant to be healed, he /she will be healed.

There are many reasons why we " get sick " or experience dis-ease. Many times it is only a message for us to stop and look at ourselves, to take the time to attune to where we are and what we are doing.

I heard a story once about a lady who was diagnosed as having breast cancer. Her doctor suggested surgery immediately. When she got the news, she had already made travel plans and was leaving within a few days. She told her doctor that when she returned from her vacation of several weeks she would schedule for surgery. Days went by and the woman really began to look at her life. She asked herself many questions. " Why do I have cancer? " " Why do I deserve this fate? " " What have I done to bring this on myself? " " Can I do anything to change this situation? " " What lessons do I need to look at in my life? "

Slowly, she began to change. Her first change was with her diet. She began eating healthier foods that were pure and natural. She learned Yoga at one of the health resorts that she visited. She began to include positive thinking and affirmations in her daily lifestyle. Day by day, week by week, step by step, the woman evolved. After her vacation ended, she returned to her doctor for another examination. The doctor ran several tests on her. No cancer could be found anywhere in her body.

Some people are not as fortunate as this woman was. For some, when they hear the call of a terminal illness, there is only a brief period of time before they leave this physical world. But for others, it is a warning to take a good look and change what needs to be changed in their lifestyles. Positive thinking, diet, loving one's self, loving others, and a reasonable exercise program have been a successful combination for many. I have witnessed and also have heard of many who have beat the terminal illness calling. If a person is meant to get well, he or she will.

Several years ago, I had a friend who was in a car accident. She hit the steering wheel with the front of her neck and it was severely traumatized. The hospital physician was contemplating doing an emergency procedure known as, a " tracheostomy ". (This is a procedure that is done to secure an airway. It invloves making an opening in the trachea (wind pipe) through the neck and a tube is inserted.) My friend was having a hard time breathing because the whole throat and neck area was severely swollen.

This situation occurred at a distance of several hundred miles from where I was residing. I was notified a short time after the accident occurred. I joined with a friend and we immediately began praying for her. We saw her whole and healthy. We projected the color vibration of green to her. It is a color of healing and balance. We also had a photograph of her that represented her presence. We sent her healing energy for about an hour and a half. I then gave the photo to my friend and he placed it in his psychotronic equipment. It runs on cosmic rays and projects this energy to the person or thing that is represented by a photo in its equipment chamber.

The next day we were notified of her successful recovery. She didn't end up needing the emergency procedure. Later on, when she was able to talk again, she informed us that she was aware of our sending her healing energy. She could feel the support and the healing changes taking place in her body. She sensed this at the exact time that it was being sent to her.

This is only a brief example. People have been helped again and again. I know of some healers who use the telephone as a tool for sending energy. The client is on one end and the healer projects energy into the phone.

I feel that some of the reasons why many are healed while others are not are for the following :

Some people choose not to be well. They are the center of everyone's attention, while they are in that physical condition. They like the attention. Many people lack love for themselves. They may have a low self-esteem and not see themselves as worthy. Some are pessimistic and enjoy others feeling sorry for them. Any of the above situations are a dead end. The cycle goes in a circle. It constantly repeats itself. They like being where they are. Even though they may be verbalizing that they want to get better, they may be giving themselves different signals on an unconscious level. Another example is that of hypochondriacs. Many have a medicine chest full of pills for any disease that their minds will create.

For many, getting well means change. Change can be a fearful thing, even if it is for our own good. Why? Because it is unfamiliar to us. This can be seen repeatedly with the elderly. The older we become, the more we begin to repeat certain patterns. We get set in our ways. We repeat what we feel works for us in our lives. It becomes familiar to us and we then find ourselves locked in a rigid structure. We create a structure of concepts, judgements and beliefs that we put in front of ourselves. We see only what we choose to see. For many, it is like putting on a pair of blinders. We get tunnel vision. We see only what is in front of us. We then lack the peripheral vision. Cosmic consciousness is all knowing and all seeing. It is an awareness that sees everything with clarity and on multiple levels all at the same time. We all have that ability within us, if we choose to aim for it. Any other consciousness is limited.

Another reason for not successfully getting well, may be based on the Law of Karma. Most metaphysicians believe that we end up in certain situations and conditions because of past actions, whether they be past actions from this life or from previous lives before this one. " You reap what you sow. " That lesson is expressed in the New Testament. The Law of Karma is the law of cause and effect, reaping what you sow.

Here are some suggestions for Absentee Healing:

Project healing color vibrations along with your prayers and meditations that you send out to those in need. Learn about Chromotherapy (Color Healing) by reading some of the books that are listed in the back of this book.

Keep a journal on Absentee Healing clients. It will help you to keep track of the following:

Time and date you sent Absentee Healings.

Supplies that you used: crystals, gemstones, essences,etc.

Methods that you used: list specific procedures or techniques.

List the physical, mental, emotional conditions of the client's initial state for your records. Also keep notes on any changes that may occur.

It helps to use photographs. If you can't obtain one, then use a signature. If you can't get either, then write down the person's name, location and age. This will be used as the " witness " to represent your client's energy vibration.

Keep a basket of tiny crystals and gemstones near your altar. These will be cleansed ahead of time, so you can use them as the need arises. I have two altars. One is for meditation. The other is for Absentee Healings and is also used on occassion for meditations.

You can place crystals and gemstones directly on the photograph or signature. This is suggested, after you become familiar with the metaphysical properties of different crystals and gemstones.

You can place a glass over the photograph or signature. The glass can be filled with water and a few drops of vibrational essences. Flower remedies, gemstone elixirs or homeopathic medicines can be put into the water. (You can use a shot glass or a small paper cup to hold the liquid.)

Dowsing Crystals can be used for clearing and projecting energy. Clear the energy by placing the pendulum over the photo or signature and let it rotate counter clockwise. It may spin for an average of one to five minutes. Visualize all negative energy being released away from the person. See the energy of the person being cleared. The pendulum will stop when it's completed. You can project energy by spinning the pendulum in a clockwise motion. If there are crystals on the photo or a cup of essences, then those energies will also be projected.

Always light candles when you do Absentee Healing work. It will remind you that your purpose is a pure one. It helps to connect you with the Divine. White, gold, purple, pink or blue candles are fine.

Trust your Inner Guidance. You will know what to do as you gain experience.

POTPOURRI

HOW TO CHARGE WATER WITH CRYSTALS

Supplies needed:

One pint or quart glass jar (The opening should be at least two inches.)

One or two small quartz crystals: Clear or Rose Quartz.

Four large Clear Quartz Crystals (palm size is good for this).

One white towel.

Center yourself into a relaxed, meditative state.

- Place small (cleansed) crystals in bottom of the jar and add non-chlorinated water.

- Go outside and find a peaceful place where you won't be disturbed. Choose a place where you can leave the crystal water to be charged for a period of time. (If you live in an apartment, you can place the jar on your patio or an open window sill that faces South where the sun shines.)

- Place the jar outside in direct sunlight on top of a white cloth or towel.

- Place four palm size crystals around all four sides of the jar. Be sure the points are directed in toward the jar. (The four crystals represent the Four Directions.)

- Do the Healing Channel Meditation. Allow yourself to center and channel healing energy. (You may also rub your hands together at this point, to activate your palm chakras.)

- Place your hands over the jar above the opening.

- Visualize healing energy going from your hands into the water and hold your hands over the jar for about three minutes. Energy follows thought. If you choose, you can visualize a particular color going into the water. You could also say an affirmation / blessing such as:
" Divine Creator, Father, Mother, Son as One bless this water. Charge this water with healing energy. May all who drink this water be blessed and filled with peace. So be it. "

- Keep the jar in direct sunlight for at least an hour. A good time is between 11:30 A.M. - 12:30 P.M. If you end up doing this procedure on a cloudy day, or in the winter time indoors, the crystals need to be in the water at least twenty-four hours.

- You can put some of the Crystal Water in a sterilized bottle with a dropper. That way it's convenient to take with you.

Most of the time, I also keep a jug of water and crystals in the refrigerator. It still works. You can taste the difference if the crystals have been in the water for at least one night. The use of distilled or Spring water is preferred over tap water. This method also works with wine. Another method for wine is to keep the closed bottle near crystals for a week.

Potpourri Notes: Crystal Uses

For women: PMS and menstrual cramps represent congested energy. Fluorite Octohedrans or Double Terminated Crystals (especially Herkimer Diamonds) are helpful in this situation. You can place them in the front pockets of your pants, or you can wear a parka with a front pocket. Keep them there as long as needed. I sometimes get intense cramps and have used either the Fluorites or Herkimers. I occasionally will place my palm chakras over the crystals and hold them in the area that feels congested or sore. Also doing the Relaxation Breath, Healing Channel Meditation or another meditation seems to help. It beats taking aspirin.

Ace wraps and crystals: When an extremity has been injured, the body will discharge positive ions. The crystals will collect these ions and help to balance out that particular area. You can place crystals inside an ace wrap, as you layer the wrap around the extremity. This helps to accelerate the healing process. Another suggestion is to use crystal pouches. You can make these or purchase them. They hold small crystals and gemstones inside the pouch. Then the pouch is placed in between the layers of the ace wrap. (The size of the minerals placed inside these pouches are the same as the ones that are used in the Absentee Healing techniques.) One combination that I used when I injured my knee once was: Clear Quartz, green Tourmaline, Amethyst and Chrysocolla. Finger size, single pointed quartz crystals can be placed along the sides of the area and a third one placed above or below the area. (This topic is discussed in more detail in the advanced classes.)

Planting Crystals

I have a friend who never had much success at growing grass in her yard. One day I suggested to her to do the following:

Cleanse a palm size Clear Quartz Crystal.

Program the crystal with the intention of it assisting the lawn in growing grass. Visualize a lot of green grass growing.

Plant the crystal in the ground in the North end of the yard. The crystal point should be aimed up towards the surface. (Quartz doesn't need to be planted very deep in the ground.) My friend planted the crystal after she seeded her lawn.

Then I also suggested that she water the lawn while she held a crystal in her LEFT hand. The other hand held the water hose. (She did the visualization that the water was helping the grass seeds to grow.)

Another suggestion was to hold the hose in her RIGHT hand and place a crystal in the path of the water. This gave her a spray effect that was similar to using a thumb to make a wider spray of the water. She then did a visualization that this crystal water was helping her grass to grow.

After a few weeks, my friend had the best grass cover on her lawn that she ever had since she had gotten her dog.

Another idea in this situation would be to use crystal water that has been charged. (See the article on " How to Charge Water with Crystals".) You could also plant four large quartz crystals in the East, South, West and North directions. Another large crystal could then be placed in the center of the lawn.

Sun Bathing with Crystals

You can make your sun bathing even more beneficial by adding crystals and gemstones to your energy field. You can do a General Layout, or the Chakra Crystal Balancing Layout, or whatever else you feel guided to do. Keep in mind that the rays of the sun will charge your crystals and you, so you'll only need a brief exposure to them.

If you do Crystal Sun Bathing at the beach, try to locate a quiet area. It doesn't help to hear loud rock and roll when you are balancing your energy. You can place the crystals in salt water when you are done. You can use a wide mouth glass jar or a plastic sand bucket for collecting the ocean water. Another suggestion is to use a fine mesh net and place your crystals inside. You can anchor this in the ocean water with a heavy stone. (This works well in a cove area.)

By doing any of the meditation exercises in this book, while Crystal Sun Bathing, your energy will be balanced more quickly. Nothing beats your own back yard or a quiet end of a park for sun bathing with crystals. Be sensitive to your own energies. You <u>can</u> overdo it.

HEALING SPACE:

CREATING THE ENVIRONMENT

When you have been doing healing work on your friends and relatives for awhile, you will reach a point of being comfortable doing it. Eventually, you may be guided to go further and become a professional. Here are some guidelines:

Select a room that is used only for healing work. It's okay if you already use the same room for meditations. You will accumulate a lot of spiritual and healing vibrations using the same environment. By keeping other influences out, you can create your own " sanctuary ". (If you can't put aside one room to be used for only spiritual work, then make do with what you have.)

When you can afford to, it is recommended to purchase a bodywork table. (See addresses at the back of this book.) For starting out you can use a chair and a foam mat. This will allow you the opportunity to alternate from using both in your session work. I scan and assess clients standing and sitting. Some of the energy work is done with the client sitting and then later, lying down on a comfortable flat surface. When purchasing a massage table, make sure your first one is a <u>lightweight</u> portable one. This will give you the freedom to take it places where you go. Massage tables average $ 350.00. You'll discover that they save on your back tremendously!

You can surround the chair with quartz crystals. If you have a massage table, you can place crystals underneath it. You can use a large Generator Crystal or some smaller ones in an energy pattern. I use a very large Amethyst crystal cluster under the table. The cluster is surrounded by a circle of Clear Quartz Crystals. The single points are pointed into the center of the circle toward the Amethyst cluster. These crystals are located beneath the upper half of the massage table.

It is also good to place crystals in each of the four corners of your Healing Room. You may use four clusters of Clear Quartz or Amethyst. Another choice would be to use four single Clear Quartz points. The points would be directed into the center of the room. You also could hang a copper pyramid over the healing table above the upper portion of the table. Some practitioners place it above the location where the client's head will be. This should be high above so the client and you don't keep bumping into it. You could attach crystals to the pyramid. (See Windows of Light by Baer.)

Next, you need a good tape player. It is a bonus to session work, if you can play mellow music. Classical: Mozart, Bach; New Age Music: any tape by Steve Halpern, Kay Gardner, or Relaxation Series, etc.

Incense is optional. Some people don't care for it. I usually burn a little, then put it out.

Sacred herbs and a burning dish, or a shell are suggested for clearing or " smudging " the environment and client. (These are recommended only for those people who are open to this kind of thing. Don't push someone's river, let it flow.)

A taper candle and holder are good for focusing and releasing into. White, blue,pink, gold or purple are nice colors to work with.

Posters are optional. I highly recommend the Chart of Your Divine Self. (We carry it.) I keep a large one in my Meditation Room and also another in my Healing Room. They are good for focusing, if you lack concentration. They are a great inspiration for the concept of channeling healing energy. Some other posters could be a Foot Reflexology chart and a Shiatsu Meridian chart.

A small shelf is nice to have for keeping some of your crystals and gemstones. This way, they can be within reach as you are guided to use them in your energy work.

A nice touch to add to the environment is a picture or two of your favorite saint or ascended master.

You now have your Healing Space. The items on the previous pages are just accessories to your work. They are not necessities.

For House Calls you may want:

- A portable massage table. (It doesn't look professional to go to your clients' homes and put them on their beds for healing work. If they are seriously ill in bed to begin with, then that's an entirely different matter.

- A suitcase with your favorite healing crystals and gemstones (see Spiritual Medicine Chest listings). Also take a candle, sacred herbs and a shell for smudging. Use only if your client and family members are open to the idea. Note: Most burnt herbs smell like marijuana smoke. I find this to be the case even with Moxibustion sticks for Shiatsu work).

- Yourself. If you don't have a table or crystals, you're fine. All you need is yourself. Anything else is just a tool for the work you already do.

The crystals and meditations are only tools to assist you in your own growth process. As you work with them, you will become more sensitive on many levels. One day you will be able to measure energy blockages with your own hands, rather than the use of the methods suggested in this book. The more you practice, the more your own healing channel will open up. Each time you explore the meditations in this book, you will go deeper inward. That is where your answers lie. The Truth lies deep within. Allow yourself to grow and expand by getting in touch with your own Inner Light.

For those who would like to go further with crystal work, I recommend many of the books listed in the back section. I have marked my favorites with an asterisk. (We usually have the popular ones in stock .) Some may desire to work closer with crystals in a " hands on " approach. We travel and offer many different workshops on Crystal Healing. I also recommend studying with other teachers. It will give you a wider exposure.

Lastly, you will learn the most about crystals from the crystals themselves.

May you grow in wisdom. PEACE.

About the Author:

REV. OJELA FRANK, M.S.C. has been active in holistic health and the healing arts for eighteen years. She has traveled extensively throughout the United States and studied many healing modalities including: Thymo-Kinesiology, Therapeutic Touch, Crystal Healing, Advanced Reiki Healing, Guided Imagery and MariEl Healing, to name a few. Ojela is an ordained Interfaith Minister and a graduate of the New Seminary in New York City. She is Director of the Holistic Health Works, which offers counseling and healing therapies. Ojela is President of Spiritual Awareness Dynamics, Inc., which offers training programs in the healing arts. Her main focus is energy balancing, counseling and teaching her clients and students how to relax and open up to their true expressions. She is author of *Crystal Basics* and is founder of the Crystal Therapeutics[sm] training seminars.

Selected Bibliography

Aebersold, Alicia. Energy Currents and Life Force. Sante Fe, N. M. : Sleeping Fox Ent., 1976.

* Alper, Frank. Exploring Atlantis Vols. I, II, III. Thousand Oaks, Ca. : Quantum Productions, 1981, 1982, 1986.

Baer, Randall & Vicki. Windows of Light. San Francisco, Ca. : Harper & Row, 1984.

Blackburn, Gabriele. The Science and Art of the Pendulum. Ojai, Ca. : Idylwild Books, 1983.

Bonewitz, Ra. Cosmic Crystals. Wellingborough, England : Turnstone Press, 1983.

Bryant, Page. Crystals and Their Use. Albuquerque, N.M. : Sun Publishing, 1984.

* Burka, Christa. Clearing Crystal Consciousness. Albuquerque, N.M. : Brotherhood of Life, 1985.

Chocron, Daya Sarai. Healing with Crystals and Gemstones. York Beach, Maine : Samuel Weiser, Inc. , 1983.

Crystal Peace. Quartz Crystals and Other Gemstones. Clyde, N.C. : Crystal Peace, 1984.

Dael. The Crystal Book. Sunol, Ca. : The Crystal Co. , 1983.

Finch, Elizabeth & Bill. Photo-Chromotherapy. Phoenix, Az. : Esoteric Publications, 1972. (out of print ?)

Gach, Michael. Acu-Yoga. New York : Japan Publications, 1981.

Gunther, Bernard. Energy Ecstasy and Your Seven Vital Chakras. Van Nuys, Ca. : Newcastle Pub.

* Gurudas. Gem Elixirs and Vibrational Healing, Vol. I. Boulder, Co. : Cassandra Press, 1985.

Hills, Christopher. Nuclear Evolution. Boulder Creek, Ca. : University of the Trees Press,1977.

Isaacs, Thelma. Gemstones, Crystals and Healing. Black Mountain, No. Carolina : Lorien House, 1982.

Joy, M.D.,Brugh. Joy's Way. L.A., Ca. : J.P. Tarcher, Inc., 1979.

* Keyes, Ken. Handbook to Higher Consciousness. Coos Bay, Or. : Ken Keyes College / Living Love Center, 1975.

* Kreiger, Dolores. The Therapeutic Touch. Engelwood Cliffs, N.J. : Prentice-Hall, Inc. , 1979.

* Kulvinskas, Victoras. Survival Into the 21st Century. Wethersfield, Conn. : Omangod Press, 1975.

Leadbeater, C.W. The Chakras. Wheaton, Ill. : Theosophical Publishing House, 1927.

Lorusso & Glick. Healing Stoned. Albuquerque, N.M. : Brotherhood of Life, 1976.

* Mariechild, Diane. Mother Wit. Trumansburg, N.Y. : The Crossing Press, 1981.

* Mickaharic, Draja. Spiritual Cleansing. York Beach, Maine : Samuel Weiser, Inc. , 1982.

Peterson, Serenity. Crystal Visioning. Nashville, Tenn. : Interdimensional Pub. , 1984.

Pough, Frederick. A Field Guide to Rocks and Minerals. Boston, Mass. : Houghton Mifflin Co. , 1953.

* Raphaell, Katrina. Crystal Enlightenment. New York : Aurora Press, 1985.

Rea, John. Healing and Quartz Crystals. Boulder, Co. : Two Trees Pub. , 1986.

Schwartz, Jack. Voluntary Controls. New York : Dutton, 1978.

Human Energy Systems. New York : Dutton, 1980.

Silbey, Uma. The Complete Crystal Guidebook. San Francisco, Ca. : U-Read Pub. , 1986.

Stewart, Nelson. Gemstones of the Seven Rays. Mokelumne Hill, Ca. : Health Research.

Richardson & Huett. Spiritual Value of Gem Stones. Marina Del Rey, Ca. : DeVorss & Co. , 1980.

Tansley, David. Chakras- Rays and Radionics. Essex, England : C.W. Daniels Co. Ltd., 1984

Tortora & Anagnostakos. Principles and Physiology. New York, N.Y. : Harper & Row, Pub., Inc. 1981.

Related Reading Material

* Anderson, Mary. Colour Healing. Wellingborough, England: Turnstone Press, 1979.

Arnold & Nevius. The Reiki Handbook. Harrisburg , Pa. : PSI Press, 1982.

Bhattacharya, A.K. Gem Therapy. Calcutta, India : Firma KLM Private Ltd, 1957.

Crow, W.B. Precious Stones. Wellingborough, England : Aquarian Press, 1968.

Campbell, Jefferson. Alive Polarity. Murrieta, Ca. : Alive Polarity Publications, 1982.

Calvery, Roger. The Healing Gems. Ottawa, Ontario, Canada : Bhakti Press, 1983.

Calvery, Roger. The Language of Crystals. Toronto, Ontario, Canada : Radionics Research Assoc. 1986.

Cayce, Edgar. Gems, Stones & Metals. Virginia Beach, Va. : Heritage Publications, 1977.

Cayce, Edgar. Gems and Stones. Virginia Beach, Va. : A.R.E. Press, 1960.

Deaver, Korra. Rock Crystal. York Beach, Maine: Samuel Weiser, Inc. 1985.

Dolfyn. Crystal Wisdom: A Beginner's Guide. Atlanta, Ga. : Blue Dolfyn Press, 1984.

Ferguson, Sibyl. The Crystal Ball. York Beach, Maine : Samuel Weiser, Inc. 1979.

Finch, Elizabeth. The Psychic Values of Gemstones. Jerome, Az. : Luminary Press, 1980.

Hodges, Doris. Healing Stones. Perry, Iowa : Pyramid Publishers of Iowa, 1961.

Jones, Alex. Seven Mansions of Color. Marina Del Rey, Ca. : DeVorss & Co., 1982.

Knopf,Alfred. The Audubon Society Field Guide to No. American Rocks and Minerals. New York: Alfred Knopf, Inc. 1978.

Kunz, George. The Curious Lore of Precious Stones. New York : Dover Publications, Inc. , 1913.

Lorusso & Glick. Stratagems: A Mineral Perspective. Albuquerque, N.M. : Brotherhood of Life, 1984.

Mariechild, Diane. Crystal Visions. Trumansburg, N.Y. : The Crossing Press, 1985.

Melville, John. Crystal Gazing and Clairvoyance. Wellingborough, England : Aquarian Press, 1979.

Miriam, Satya. The Healing Power of Gemstones. Berkeley, Ca.

Mohring, Martha. The Serpent and the Stone. Rialto, Ca. : SanGraal Press, 1984.

Rendel. Peter. Introduction to the Chakras. Wellingborough, England : Acquarian Press, 1974.

Saha, N.N. Healing Through Gems. New Delhi, India : Sterling Publishers Private Ltd. , 1984.

Smith, Michael. Crystal Power. St. Paul, Minn. : LLewellyn Pub. , 1985.

Tansley, David. Subtle Body. New York, N.Y. : Thames & Hudson, 1977.

Uyldert, Mellie. The Magic of Precious Stones. Wellingborough, England: Turnstone Press, 1981.

Recommended Readings

Auel, Jean. Clan of the Cave Bear. New York : Bantam Books.
Baker, Douglas. Esoteric Healing. Herts, England, 1975.
Blum, Ralph. The Book of Runes. New York : St. Martin's Press, 1982.
Burke, Abbot George. Magnetic Therapy. Okla. City, Ok.: St. George, 1980.
Emery, Stewart. Actualizations. New York: Doubleday, 1978.
Foundation For Inner Peace. A Course In Miracles. Tiburon, Ca., 1975.
Gawain,Shakti. Creative Visualization. New York : Bantam Books, 1982.
Gennaro, Guzzon & Marsigli. Kirlian Photography. London : East/West, 1980.
Gordon, Richard. Your Healing Hands. Santa Cruz, Ca. : Unity Press, 1978.
Hauschka, Margarethe. Rhythmical Massage. London : Rudolf Steiner Press, 1979. (out of print).
Hay, Louise. Heal Your Body. Santa Monica, Ca. : Hay House, 1982.
Heline, Corinne. Healing and Regeneration Through Color. Marina Del Rey, Ca. : DeVorss & Co., 1980.
Holmes, Ernest. The Science of Mind. New York : Dodd, Mead & Co. , 1938.
Hunt, Roland. The Seven Keys to Color Healing. San Francisco, Ca. : Harper & Row, 1971.
Jampolsky M.D. , Gerald. Love Is Letting Go Of Fear. New York : Bantam Books, 1979.
Johari, Harish. Dhanwantari. San Francisco, Ca. : Rams Head Inc., 1974.
Kroeger, Hannah. Magneto-Therapy : the Laying on of Hands. Boulder, Co.
Kueshana, Eklal. The Ultimate Frontier. Stelle, Ill. : The Stelle Group, 1970.
Levi. The Aquarian Gospel of Jesus the Christ. Marina Del Rey, Ca. : DeVorss & Co. , 1907.
Levine, Stephen. A Gradual Awakening. New York : Doubleday, 1979.
Miller, Roberta. Psychic Massage. San Francisco, Ca. : Harper & Row, 1975.
Moody M.D. , Raymond. Life After Life. New York : Bantam Books, 1975.
Newman & Berkowitz. How To Be Your Own Best Friend. New York : Ballantine Books, 1971.
Noud van den Eerenbeemt. Divination By Magic. York Beach, Maine : Samuel Weiser Inc., 1982.
Ouseley, S.G.J. The Power of the Rays. Essex, England : Fowler & Co., 1951.
Ouseley, S.G.J. Colour Meditations. Essex, England : Fowler & Co., 1949.

Prophet, Elizabeth Clare. The Lost Years of Jesus. Malibu, Ca. : Summit Univ. Press, 1984.

Rogat, Steven. Magnetic Therapy & Its Application to the Menstrual Cycle. Colorado Springs, Colo. , 1982.

Roquemore, Kathleen. It's All in Your Numbers. New York : Harper & Row, 1975.

Shain, Merle. Some Men Are More Perfect Than Others. New York : Bantam Books, 1973.

Sherwood, Keith. The Art of Spiritual Healing. St. Paul, Minn. : Llewellyn Pub., 1985.

Steiner, Rudolf. Knowledge of the Higher Worlds and Its Attainment. New York : Anthroposophic Press, Inc. 1961.

Szekely, Edmond B. The Essene Gospel of Peace.

—————. The Discovery of the Essene Gospel of Peace. Cartago, Costa Rica, Central America : I.B.S. Internacional, 1937.

Two Disciples. The Rainbow Bridge. Escondido, Ca. : The Triune Foundation, 1981.

Williams, Anne The Pendulum Book of Charts. New York : Pendulums Plus 1979.

Wydro, Kenneth. Flying Solo. New York : Berkley Books, 1979.

EXPANDING YOUR HORIZONS

Metaphysical Conferences

Medicine Wheel Gatherings

Contact : Singing Pipe Woman, (509) 326-6561.
The Bear Tribe Medicine Society
Box 9167
Spokane, Wash. 99209

(Native American traditions, Medicine Wheel, sweat lodges, workshops).

Spiritual Frontier Fellowship

Contact : Spiritual Frontier Fellowship - National Headquarters
10819 Winner Rd.
Independence, Mo. 64052

Spiritual Frontier Fellowship - North East Retreat
Diane Downer, Register
167 Warren Way
Lancaster, Penna. 17601

(National and regional seminars, workshops on healing and metaphysics).

Waldorf Institute

Contact : Waldorf Institue
Hungry Hollow Rd.
Spring Valley, N.Y. 10977

(Teachings of Rudolf Steiner - Anthroposophy, Spiritual Science, healing, Biodynamics, Waldorf Education schools, special communities around the world).

Life Spectrums

Contact : Life Spectrums - North East Region
P.O.Box 373
Harrisburg, Pa. 17108

Life Spectrums - Canada Conference
Carol Tucker, Register
2177 Lincoln Ave. #18
Montreal, P.Q., Canada, H3H1J2

(Conferences and workshops on healing and metaphysics).

The American Society of Dowsers, Inc.

Contact : The American Society of Dowsers, Inc.
Danville, Vermont 05828

(Seminars, dowsing information and supplies).

Healing Training Seminars

Reiki Healing Seminars

Contact : The Reiki Alliance
535 Cordova Rd. Suite 419
Santa Fe, New Mexico 87501
(505) 983-8659

(International seminars, certification for practitioners and teaching).

Therapeutic Touch

Contact : Institute of Integrative Nursing, Div. of Nursing
New York University
429 Shimkin Hall, Washingtion Sq.
New York, N.Y. 10003
(212) 598-3921

(Courses in Therapeutic Touch and alternative nursing).

Pumpkin Hollow Farm
R.R. 1 Box 135
Craryville, N.Y. 12521

(Summer training programs in Therapeutic Touch).

Crystal Healing Seminars

Contact : Crystal Therapeutics[SM]
P.O. Box 596, Dept. C.B.
Bardonia, N.Y. 10954
(914) 634-2450

(National seminars and certification training).

MariEl Healing Seminars

Contact : Ethel Lombardi
93 Spring Creek Rd. Rte. 5
Lockport, Ill. 60441
(815) 838-8218

(National seminars and certification training).

Organizations

American Holistic Nurses Association
P.O. Box 116
Telluride, Colo. 81435

(Membership open to all nurses, newsletters, local and area network groups, speakers bureau, and regional / national conferences).

Nurse Healers Professional Assoc., Inc.
c/o Membership Committee
1827 Haight Street, Suite 157
San Francisco, Ca. 94117

(Membership open to nurses and health care providers with a mininum Bachelors Degree. National / regional support groups, lectures, newsletters, and conferences).

Retreats & Seminars

Omega Institute
Lake Drive
R.D. 2 Box 377
Rhinebeck, N.Y. 12572
(914) 338-6030 until May / (914) 266-4301 summer camp.

(Week and weekend seminars during the summer).

Kripalu Center
Box 793
Lenox, Mass. 01240

(A retreat center for mind, body and spirit with certification training in healing, bodywork and yoga).

Rainbow Gathering Festivals

Rainbow Family Tribal
P.O. Box 323
Plymouth Meeting, Pa. 19462

(New Age group gatherings that network on regional and national levels.)

Assoc. for Research and Enlightenment
P.O. Box 595
Virginia Beach, Va. 23451
(804) 428-3588

(ARE, founded by Edgar Cayce in 1931, seminars in healing and spiritual growth).

Brugh Joy, Inc.
P.O. Box 895
Lucerne Valley, Ca. 92356
(619) 247-5651

(Healing seminars and teachings based on the book, Joy's Way).

Metaphysical Tours

Healing the Earth Ceremonial Tours

Dr. Joe Jochmans
c/o World Light Travels, Inc.
P.O. Box 9508
Wyoming, Mich. 49509
(616) 531-1339)

also:

c/o Holistic Life Travels
P.O. Box 478
Fairfax, Ca. 94930
(415) 459-8070

(Dr. Jochmans, author of <u>Rolling Thunder : The Coming of the Earth Changes</u> is one of the <u>best</u> metaphysical tour guides in the world. Trips to: Peru, Ancient Egypt, Ancient Greece, Hawaii, Mexico, Arthurian England, and Ancient Israel. Trips include: visitations to ancient ruins, group meditations, archealogical and metaphysical explanations of ancient civilizations, planetary healing with crystals and powerful ceremonial initiations.)

Psychic Surgeons of the Phillipines

Rev. Margie Laird
c/o Vega International Travel Service, Inc.
201 N. Wells St.
Chicago, Ill. 60606
(312) 332-7211)

(Advance healing seminars which include: studying with famous Phillipine healers. Rev. Laird has been a tour guide to the Phillipines for over fifteen years. She is also a famous healer in the Wilmington, Dela. area.)

For Expanding Your Holistic Practice

Products for healing and self-growth:

Contact : Holistic Health Works
P.O. Box 327-CTB
New City, N.Y. 10956 USA.
(914) 634-2450

Bodywork supplies, quartz crystals, clusters, gemstones, mineral specimens, crystal energy jewelry, gem elixirs, flower remedies, oils, homeopathic medicines, Native American supplies, books, Dowsing Crystals, relaxation music tapes, video tapes on healing and New Age teachings, energy tools, meditation supplies. (Retail and Wholesale).

Bodywork Tables

Living Earth Crafts
600 E. Todd Rd.
Santa Rosa, Ca. 95407
(800) 358-8292 or in Calif. (800) 336-4114

Oakworks, Inc.
1306 Rayville Rd.
Parkton, Md. 21120
(800) 558-8850

Golden Ratio Woodworks
P.O. Box 297
Emigrant, Mt. 59027
(800) 345-1129

Robert Hunter - Bodywork Tables
1104 N.E. 28th
Portland, Oregon 97232
(503) 249-0847

New Age Periodicals

East/West Journal
P.O. Box 1200
Brookline, Mass. 02147

Gnosis Magazine
The Lumen Foundation
P.O. Box 14217
San Francisco, Ca. 94114

Magical Blend
P.O. Box 11303
San Francisco, 94101

Massage Magazine
Box 1969
Kealakekua, Hawaii 96750

Mothering Magazine
Mothering Publications
P.O. Box 8410
Santa Fe, New Mexico 87504

New Age Journal
342 Western Ave.
Brighton, Mass. 02135

Shaman's Drum
P.O. Box 2636
Berkeley, Ca. 94702

Wildfire Magazine
The Bear Tribe Medicine Society
Box 9167
Spokane, Wash. 99209

Yoga Journal
P.O. Box 15203
Santa Ana, Ca. 92705

NOTES ON MY CRYSTAL EXPERIENCES: